ANATOMY & 100 ESSENTIAL STRETCHING EXERCISES FOR

Tennis

and other racket sports, including paddleball, squash, and badminton

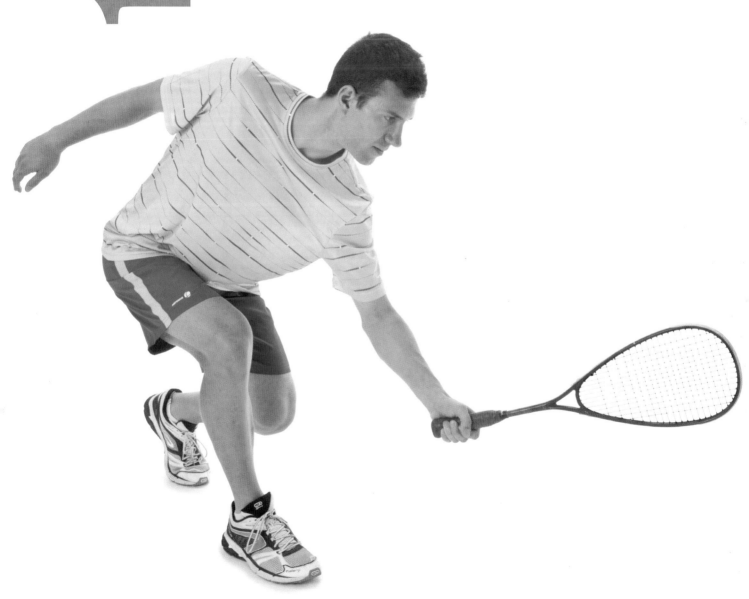

BARRON'S

ANATOMY & ESSENTIAL STRETCHING

100 EXERCISES FOR

Tennis

and other racket sports, including paddleball, squash, and badminton

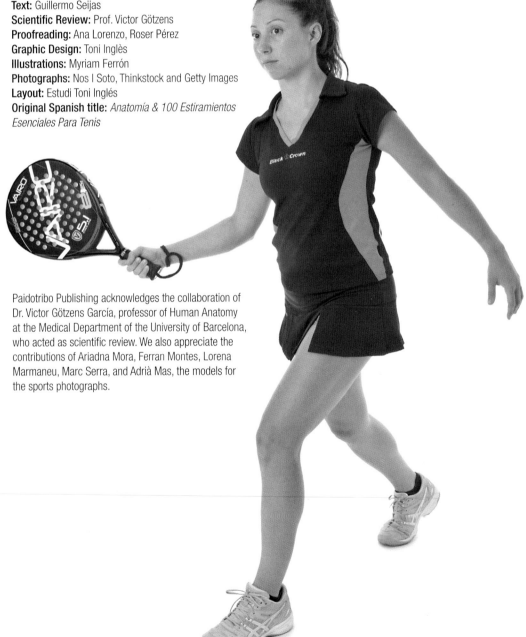

Editorial Director: María Fernanda Canal
Text: Guillermo Seijas
Scientific Review: Prof. Victor Götzens
Proofreading: Ana Lorenzo, Roser Pérez
Graphic Design: Toni Inglès
Illustrations: Myriam Ferrón
Photographs: Nos I Soto, Thinkstock and Getty Images
Layout: Estudi Toni Inglés
Original Spanish title: *Anatomía & 100 Estiramientos Esenciales Para Tenis*

First edition for the United States, its territories and dependencies, and Canada published in 2017 by Barron's Educational Series, Inc.

English-language translation © copyright 2017 by Barron's Educational Series, Inc. English translation by Eric A. Bye, M.A.

© Copyright 2017 by Editorial Paidotribo—World Rights Published by Editorial Paidotribo, Badalona, Spain

All inquiries should be addressed to:
Barron's Educational Series, Inc.
250 Wireless Boulevard
Hauppauge, NY 11788
www.barronseduc.com

ISBN: 978-1-4380-0969-8

Library of Congress Control No.:
  2016946250

Printed in Spain
9 8 7 6 5 4 3 2 1

Paidotribo Publishing acknowledges the collaboration of Dr. Victor Götzens García, professor of Human Anatomy at the Medical Department of the University of Barcelona, who acted as scientific review. We also appreciate the contributions of Ariadna Mora, Ferran Montes, Lorena Marmaneu, Marc Serra, and Adrià Mas, the models for the sports photographs.

Preface

You probably had your first experience with racket and paddle sports when you were very young. Most of us have played paddleball at the beach, in the park, or in school, using some rudimentary implement, perhaps of plastic or wood, to hit a ball and send it off like a shot.

Perhaps later on you forgot this sensation and left this type of sport behind until one day, without knowing how, you found yourself interested once again in tennis, badminton, paddleball, or other racket sports. Or perhaps you never gave up your racket sport and now you are an advanced player or even a veteran who is starting to feel the effects of so many hours of play.

Whatever the case, there is still plenty of road ahead of you, whether to improve your game, to get over any discomfort resulting from your activity, or both. The issue is being able to continue enjoying one or more of these sports, sharing the time with your friends, and especially, doing it in full measure.

In this sense it is appropriate to know the various factors that will determine your capacity to face the game and enjoy it. These include everything from the equipment, which must be selected in accordance with your abilities and your characteristics as a player, to the proper training to participate in matches with physical and technical security, considering any injuries you may have experienced in the past or that you hope to prevent. Managing these factors will certainly work to your advantage and make you a more competent player on the court, with greater knowledge of your hobby and lower risk of suffering sports injuries that could impact your daily life.

Nothing should keep athletes, whether occasional or regular, from their hobby, and any opportunity to deepen their knowledge should be seen as a window to improvement, and as a challenge to be met in enjoying healthy, active leisure time.

These pages present answers to many of the questions that you may have had about your sport at some time; they will show you the effects on your body and ways to prepare it—all in a clear, intuitive manner. See for yourself and start getting the most out of your playing.

Contents

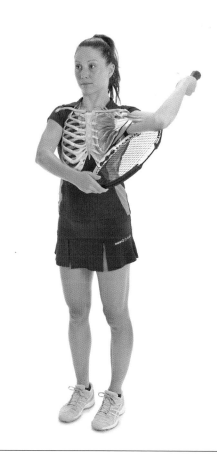

How to Use This Book

Number of
the stretch

Name of the
stretch

Area
worked

Muscle
stretched

IDENTIFICATION
OF THE STRETCH

PERFORMANCE OF
THE STRETCH

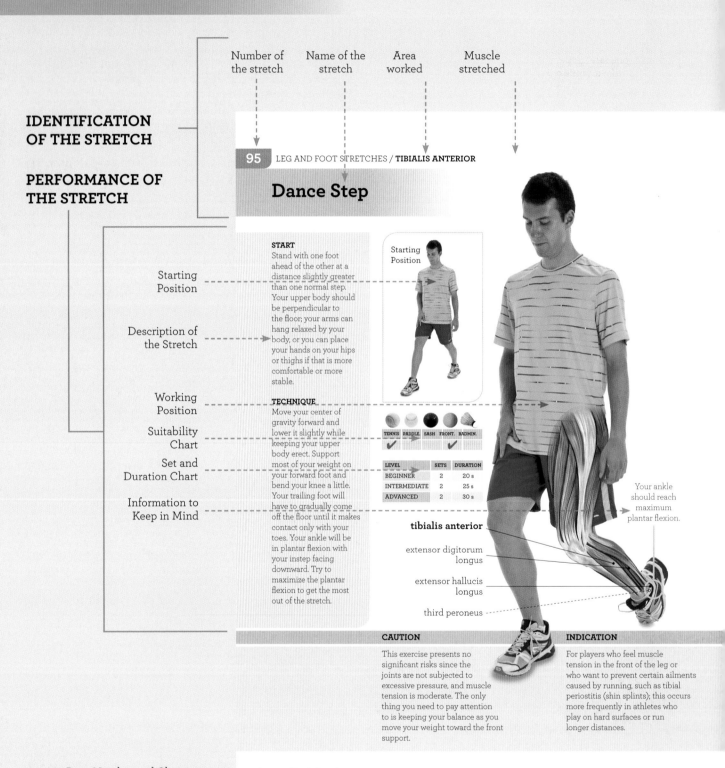

95 LEG AND FOOT STRETCHES / **TIBIALIS ANTERIOR**

Dance Step

Starting
Position

Starting
Position

START
Stand with one foot
ahead of the other at a
distance slightly greater
than one normal step.
Your upper body should
be perpendicular to
the floor; your arms can
hang relaxed by your
body, or you can place
your hands on your hips
or thighs if that is more
comfortable or more
stable.

Description of
the Stretch

TECHNIQUE
Move your center of
gravity forward and
lower it slightly while
keeping your upper
body erect. Support
most of your weight on
your forward foot and
bend your knee a little.
Your trailing foot will
have to gradually come
off the floor until it makes
contact only with your
toes. Your ankle will be
in plantar flexion with
your instep facing
downward. Try to
maximize the plantar
flexion to get the most
out of the stretch.

Working
Position

Suitability
Chart

Set and
Duration Chart

Information to
Keep in Mind

	TENNIS	PADDLE.	SASH	FRONT.	BADMIN.
	✔			✔	

LEVEL	SETS	DURATION
BEGINNER	2	20 s
INTERMEDIATE	2	25 s
ADVANCED	2	30 s

Your ankle
should reach
maximum
plantar flexion.

tibialis anterior

extensor digitorum
longus

extensor hallucis
longus

third peroneus

CAUTION
This exercise presents no
significant risks since the
joints are not subjected to
excessive pressure, and muscle
tension is moderate. The only
thing you need to pay attention
to is keeping your balance as you
move your weight toward the front
support.

INDICATION
For players who feel muscle
tension in the front of the leg or
who want to prevent certain ailments
caused by running, such as tibial
periostitis (shin splints); this occurs
more frequently in athletes who
play on hard surfaces or run
longer distances.

Page Number and Chapter **144** / Static Stretches

one stretch per page,
like an index card

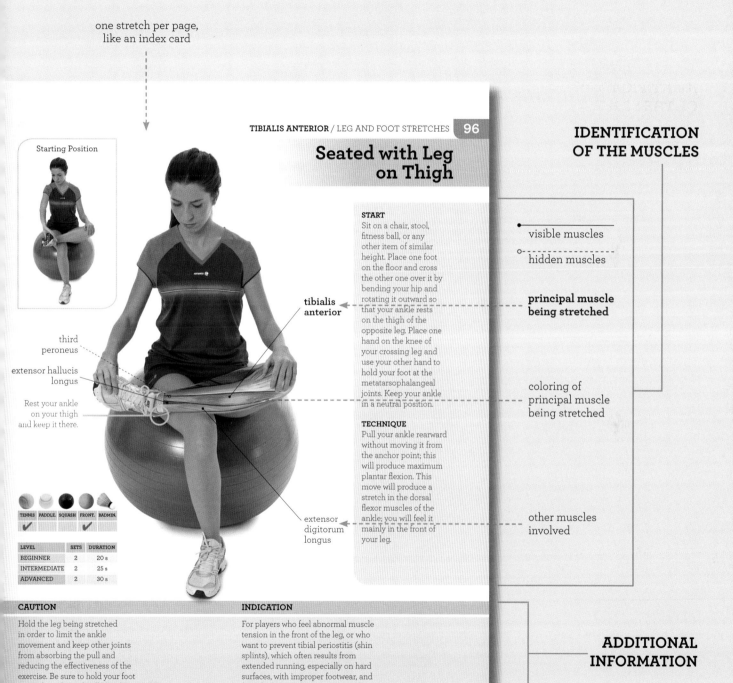

Starting Position

Seated with Leg on Thigh

START
Sit on a chair, stool, fitness ball, or any other item of similar height. Place one foot on the floor and cross the other one over it by bending your hip and rotating it outward so that your ankle rests on the thigh of the opposite leg. Place one hand on the knee of your crossing leg and use your other hand to hold your foot at the metatarsophalangeal joints. Keep your ankle in a neutral position.

TECHNIQUE
Pull your ankle rearward without moving it from the anchor point; this will produce maximum plantar flexion. This move will produce a stretch in the dorsal flexor muscles of the ankle; you will feel it mainly in the front of your leg.

tibialis anterior

third peroneus

extensor hallucis longus

Rest your ankle on your thigh and keep it there.

extensor digitorum longus

TENNIS	PADDLE.	SQUASH	FRONT.	BADMIN.
✔			✔	

LEVEL	SETS	DURATION
BEGINNER	2	20 s
INTERMEDIATE	2	25 s
ADVANCED	2	30 s

IDENTIFICATION OF THE MUSCLES

• visible muscles

○ hidden muscles

principal muscle being stretched

coloring of principal muscle being stretched

other muscles involved

CAUTION
Hold the leg being stretched in order to limit the ankle movement and keep other joints from absorbing the pull and reducing the effectiveness of the exercise. Be sure to hold your foot correctly and avoid pulling it by the toes.

INDICATION
For players who feel abnormal muscle tension in the front of the leg, or who want to prevent tibial periostitis (shin splints), which often results from extended running, especially on hard surfaces, with improper footwear, and from fairly long distances covered.

ADDITIONAL INFORMATION

Anatomical Atlas
Locations of the Muscles

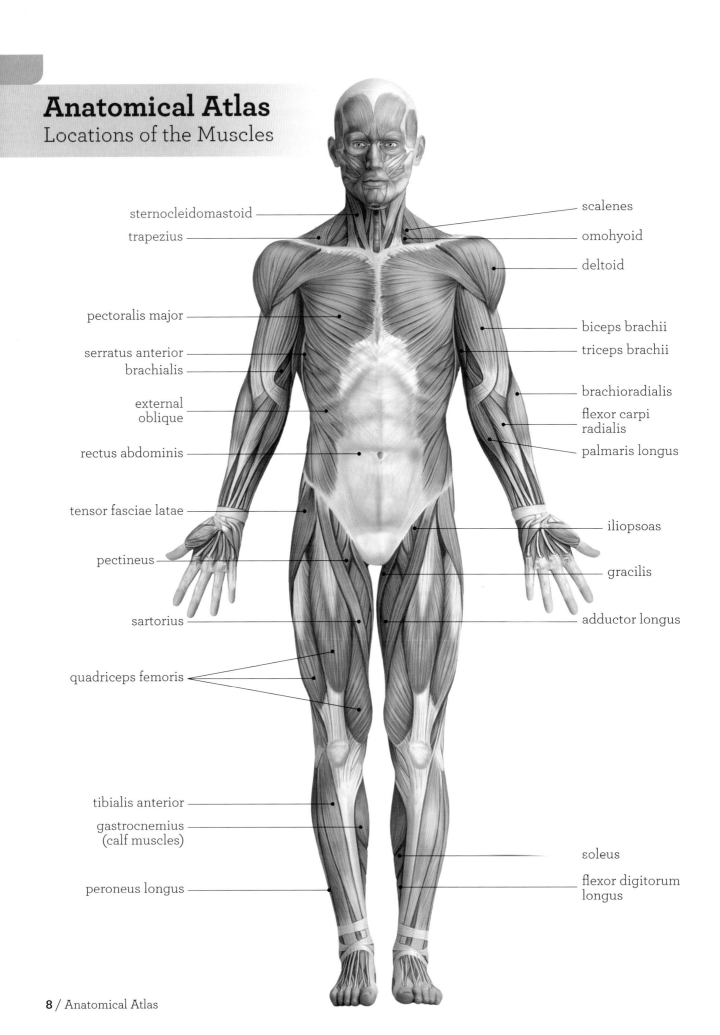

sternocleidomastoid

trapezius

pectoralis major

serratus anterior

brachialis

external oblique

rectus abdominis

tensor fasciae latae

pectineus

sartorius

quadriceps femoris

tibialis anterior

gastrocnemius (calf muscles)

peroneus longus

scalenes

omohyoid

deltoid

biceps brachii

triceps brachii

brachioradialis

flexor carpi radialis

palmaris longus

iliopsoas

gracilis

adductor longus

soleus

flexor digitorum longus

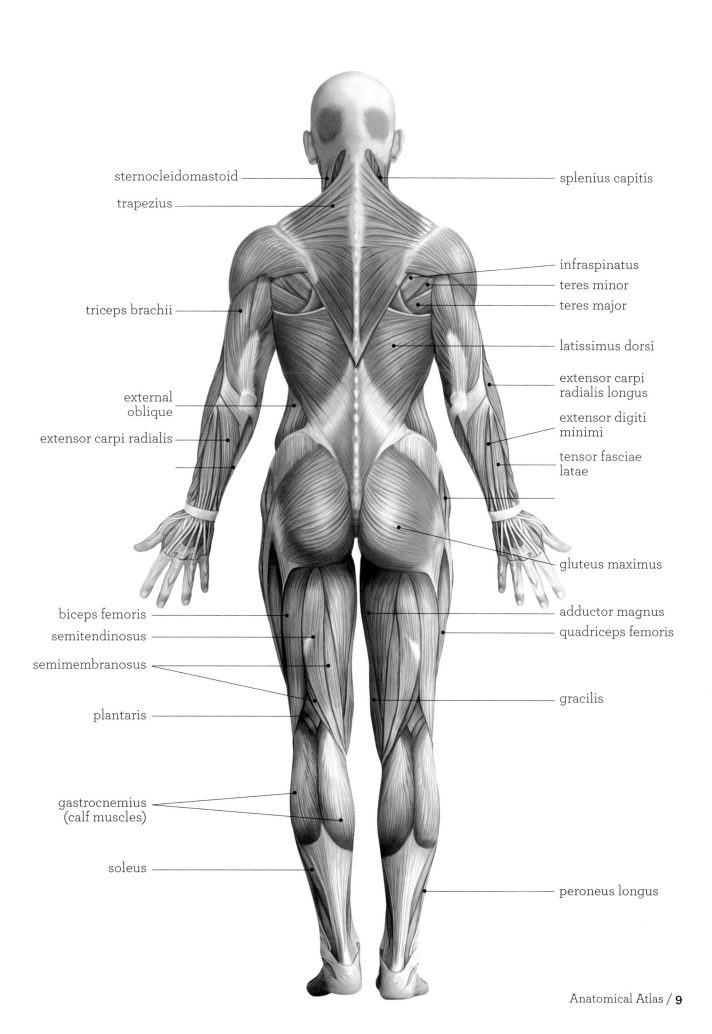

sternocleidomastoid

trapezius

triceps brachii

external
oblique

extensor carpi radialis

biceps femoris

semitendinosus

semimembranosus

plantaris

gastrocnemius
(calf muscles)

soleus

splenius capitis

infraspinatus

teres minor

teres major

latissimus dorsi

extensor carpi
radialis longus

extensor digiti
minimi

tensor fasciae
latae

gluteus maximus

adductor magnus

quadriceps femoris

gracilis

peroneus longus

Planes of Movement

Before we start, it is necessary to explain a series of terms that refer to body movements, and which appear in recurring fashion throughout the book. If you do not know the basic nomenclature of the movements it will be difficult to understand the detailed descriptions of the exercises. Some of these terms, such as *bending* and *extending* are in common usage, but others, such as *inversion*, *eversion*, *adduction*, and *supination*, are often used in narrower circles, so it may be very useful to review their meaning.

The first thing we need to know is that body movements take place in three different planes: the frontal, the sagittal, and the transverse planes. There is a certain group of movements that correspond to each plane, as we will see below. We can begin to understand them with the basic anatomical position in the illustration.

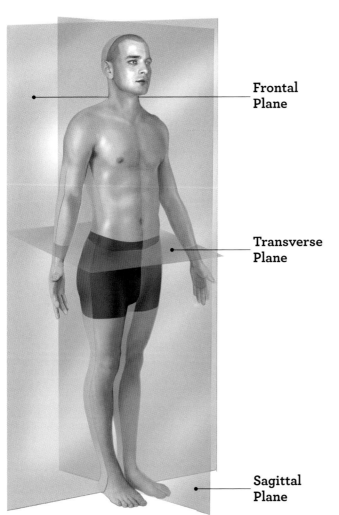

Frontal Plane

Transverse Plane

Sagittal Plane

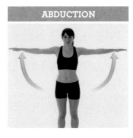
ABDUCTION

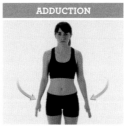
ADDUCTION

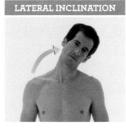
LATERAL INCLINATION

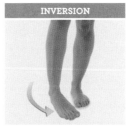
INVERSION

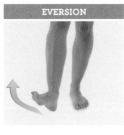
EVERSION

FRONTAL PLANE

This divides the body into a ventral and a dorsal part; in other words, front and back. The chest and the stomach are in the ventral plane, and the back of the neck, the back, and the buttocks are in the dorsal part. The movements in the frontal plane are as follows:

Abduction: a movement in which we move a limb away from the central axis of the body. This is easily seen from the front or the rear, since the variation in the outline of the body is easy to see from this perspective. When we hold our arms straight out to the side we perform abduction of the shoulders.

Adduction: a movement in which we bring a limb toward the central axis of the body; in other words, the movement opposite abduction. If we stand with our arms straight out to the side and we lower them so they are close to our body, we perform adduction of the shoulders.

Lateral Inclination: a movement in which we tilt our head, our neck, or our upper body to the side. If we fall asleep in a sitting position, generally our head and neck end up tipping to one side through lateral inclination.

Inversion: Although this movement does not belong solely to the frontal plane, this is where it is most common. Foot inversion occurs when the toes and the sole are moved toward the inside while performing plantar flexion.

Eversion: a turning movement toward the outside; for example, the toes and the sole of the foot face outward while performing dorsal flexion.

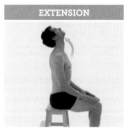

FLEXION

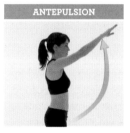

EXTENSION

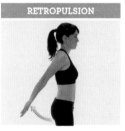

ANTEPULSION

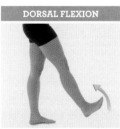

RETROPULSION

DORSAL FLEXION

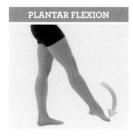

PLANTAR FLEXION

SAGITTAL PLANE

This divides the body into two halves: right and left. Movements in this plane are best perceived by looking at the individual's profile from one side. The following movements are clearly visible in this plane:

Flexion: a movement in which we move one part of the body ahead with respect to the central axis. There are exceptions to this definition, such as knee flexion and plantar flexion of the ankle.

Extension: a movement in which we move a part of the body rearward with respect to the central axis, or we align it with the axis. For example, if we stand and look up at the sky, we have to perform an extension of the cervical vertebrae. Once again, the knee is an exception.

Antepulsion: This is equivalent to flexion, but it is applicable solely to the movement of the shoulder.

Retropulsion: This is equivalent to extension, but it is applicable solely to the movement of the shoulder.

Dorsal Flexion: a flexion movement that is applicable solely to the ankle joint.

Plantar Flexion: the term used to designate the ankle movement equivalent to extension.

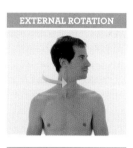

EXTERNAL ROTATION

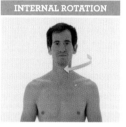

INTERNAL ROTATION

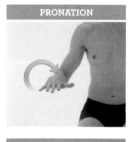

PRONATION

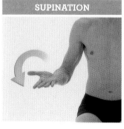

SUPINATION

TRANSVERSE PLANE

This divides the body into an upper and a lower part. Movements in this plane are easily seen from any vantage point, although somewhat better from above or below the individual. They are as follows:

External Rotation: a movement in which we turn a body part toward the outside and along its axis. If we are seated at a table and the person next to us speaks to us, we perform an external rotation of the neck to look at him as he speaks.

Internal Rotation: a movement opposite the previous one, since it involves turning a part of the body toward the inside along its axis. When we complete the conversation with the person sitting next to us, we perform an internal rotation of the neck to return our gaze toward the front.

Pronation: a rotational movement of the forearm, in which we place the back of the hand upward and the palm facing downward. When we use a knife or a fork to manipulate the food on a plate, our hands are in pronation.

Supination: a movement opposite the previous one, which involves rotating the forearm in such a way that we place the palms facing upward. For example, if someone gives us a handful of sunflower seeds, we place our hands palms-up, in supination, similar to a bowl, so we don't drop them.

A Brief History of Racket Sports

It is no easy task to determine the ultimate origin of the paddle and racket sports. In the history of sports, all kinds of games and physical and sporting activities intersect, mix with one another, and even end up disappearing or turning into familiar disciplines.

Some of the ball games of which we have records were played thousands of years ago. From the Beni Hassan tomb inscriptions dating from some four thousand years ago, we know that in ancient Egypt small-size balls were used in doing various physical fitness exercises, including juggling. Also at the temple of Ramesses III, there are carvings relating to ball games and other disciplines that could be done for recreation or military training.

In classical Greece, ball games likewise played a prominent role as a basic component of training for children and adolescents, as well as entertainment for adult men and women. They were part of their culture, and there are references to them in the *Odyssey* by Homer. Still the ancient Greeks did not give these practices the importance that they devoted to track and wrestling events, and they were not part of the great competitions such as the original Olympic Games. Some carved representations of these games have come down to us, but the limited depictions do not allow us to know precisely what they were like. But we still know that there were games such as *aporraxis*, where the object was to throw a ball hard against the ground; *episkyros*, in which the ball was thrown at the opponent's playing field in an attempt to capture territory; *trigon*, in which a ball was passed among three players on the field so that they marked the three vertices of a triangle; and *urania*, in which the players sought to catch a ball thrown into the air. There is evidence of games that may have resembled current-day pelota and frontenis, since the object was to bounce the ball against a wall.

Various types of ball games also were played during the Roman Empire. At that time, physical and sporting events were often, though not exclusively, related to religious celebrations. Some of the games came from classical Greece, such as *trigon* and *urania*, and they were played in a similar way. In other cases, as with *harpastum*, the original game had undergone significant changes, and physical contact was allowed, turning it into a tough game similar to today's rugby, so often this was considered part of military training. In addition, and even though the Romans did not use rackets or similar implements, blows with the hand to keep the ball from falling to the ground turned into a regular practice in some games, including *ludus pilae cum palma*.

In various cultures of pre-Columbian America people also played ball games as religious celebrations. More than 3,000 years ago in Mesoamerica the first recorded rituals in this part of the world that included ball games took place. More than a dozen variants of these games are known, most of which were played with oilskin balls made of rubber from a tree that is widespread in Central and South America. In general, two teams faced one another in an attempt to send the ball toward the rival field. The ball had to remain in the air as long as possible, and depending

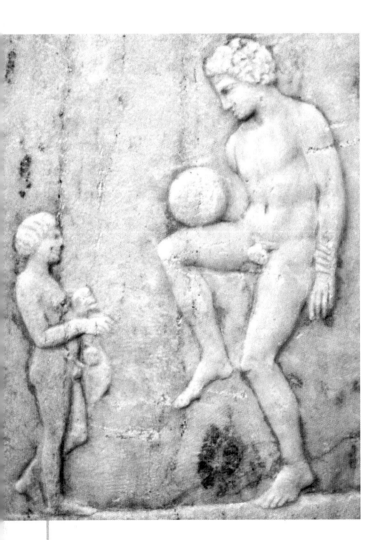

Marble bas-relief from classical Greece showing a ball game.

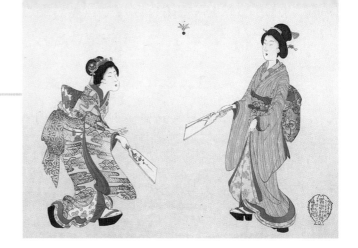

Representation of the traditional Japanese game hanetsuki.

on the variant of the game, the players could hit it with their knees, hips, elbows, and forearms, gauntlets, or various implements. It is believed that the ball was assigned an astrological meaning: it may have represented the sun or the moon, and its movements in the air imitated its motion through the heavens. The best known of these games was *tlatchtli*, played in a court with leaning or vertical side walls and two stone rings that the ball was supposed to hit or pass through. There are still several places in existence that were constructed specifically for playing these ritual games, including the one at Chichén-Itzá, which was built by the Mayas. We know that these practices were closely linked to human sacrifices, but there is still controversy over whether the sacrifice was a punishment for the losers or an honor for the winners.

As early as the fourth century B.C. the Persians were playing *tchigan*, the first known game involving the use of instruments that could be called rackets. This primitive racket was made of wood and had strings that probably were made from gut or plant materials strong enough for hitting the ball. This game spread, with variations, through Asia, and we have references to racket games in China,

Japan, and India, although no clear relationship among them can be established.

In ancient times many other games were played that retain some connection to present-day racket and paddle games, but they could not be presented in a single book. A list of all the games that attained a certain social relevance would fill hundreds of pages, without mentioning the thousands of popular local games that could have been the true ancestors of today's tennis, squash, and badminton. Thus we will focus on finding a more modern origin that provides more references about our current racket and paddle sports.

If there is one game that cannot be overlooked because of its indisputable influence on current-day racket and paddle sports, it is the *jeu de paume*, which goes back about a thousand years. It was surely

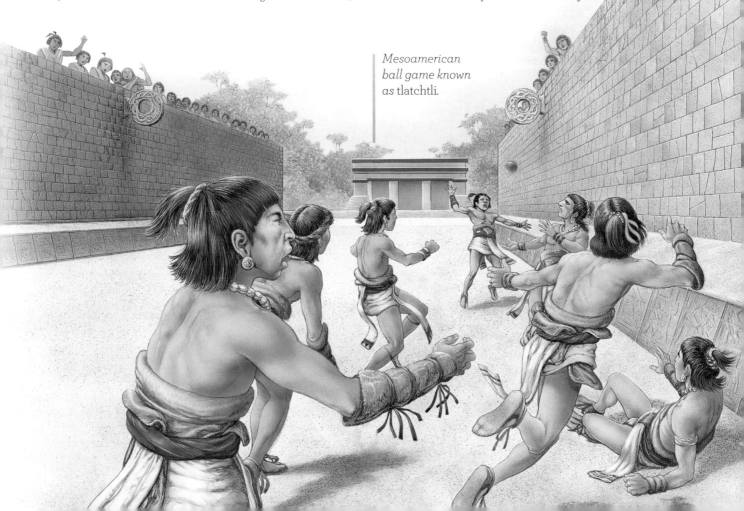

Mesoamerican ball game known as tlatchtli.

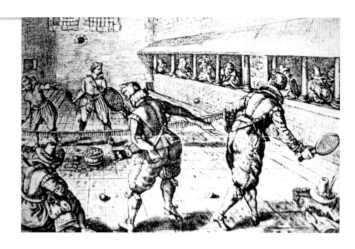

Engraving showing a jeu de paume *match.*

of European origin, and although a similar version was played in some religious communities in France as early as the 11th century, it is certain that Paris was the city in which this game was most influential. In the *jeu de paume*, two or more contestants divided into two teams used their hands to strike a small ball made of skin to make it fly over a suspended tape, rope, or cord that was the dividing line between the playing areas of the two teams or contestants. Early on there were two versions of the game: the *longue paume*, which was played outdoors, and the *courte paume*, which took place in closed spaces. The latter version was played in halls enclosed by walls that caused the ball to bounce. This feature allowed for more continuous play since the ball could not escape through the ends or the sides of the playing area, and the players had more opportunities for returns. Also the surface underfoot generally was smoother, so it was easier to predict the bounce, and people could play regardless of weather conditions.

Little by little, modifications were introduced, including the gradual abandonment using the hand, due mainly to the rough nature of the game, and the adoption of a type of gauntlet that protected the hand, and then paddles, and finally rackets. As the game gained more recognition and the number of adherents increased, more money became associated with it: betting and professional players came into being, and special halls were built, and some artisans specialized in making rackets and balls, among other things. In Paris at the end of the 16th century there were 250 *jeu de paume* courts and about a dozen artisans who made balls, and because of the quality their reputation extended beyond the French borders.

In England this same game was known under the name of *royal tennis*, and it spread through the rest of Europe, although with different names and various differences in the regulations.

This game surely was the precursor of modern tennis, and probably of other activities such as paddleball, squash, and frontenis, although, as we will see later one, there are other points in history that bring us closer to each of these sports.

One of the hypotheses that supports the possibility that Reverend Frank Peer Baal was the one who, at the end of the 19th century, in his desire to adapt tennis to smaller players, modified the dimensions of the court and replaced the racket with a paddle and used balls with lower pressure to control the bounce; this may have given rise to modern paddle tennis, a game that in turn could be the precursor of platform tennis and paddleball.

The International Paddleball Federation maintains that the inventor of this sport was the impresario Enrique

Corcuera; using a plot of land at his house in Acapulco, and taking inspiration from paddle tennis, which he had played, he built a court with walls almost ten feet (3 m) tall at the ends and slightly lower at the sides and began playing a game with a paddle that eventually evolved into modern paddleball.

Mexico was also the birthplace of frontenis, a combination of some features of tennis and Basque pelota, at the start of the 20th century.

As for squash, it seems that in the early 19th century, during the heyday of racket sports, prisoners in London's Fleet Prison began hitting a ball and bouncing it off the prison walls. Despite its strange place of origin, it didn't take long for this game to jump over the walls that confined it, and soon it was played in English schools, including Harrow, where it was called *rackets*. Here it gained popularity, and people began using balls with less bounce to intensify the game and force the players to run

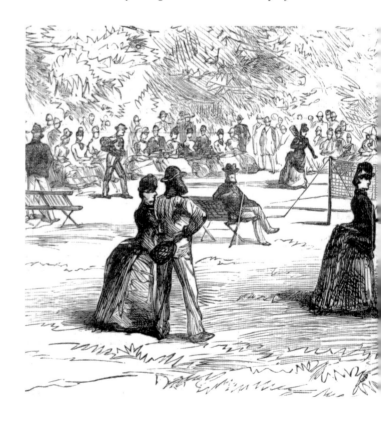

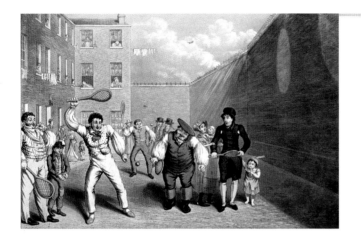

after the ball instead of waiting for it to come back to them after bouncing off the wall. That was the birth of a new and popular form that turned into modern-day squash.

Finally, we should note the possible origins of badminton. It seems that as early as the Middle Ages people played *battledore and shuttlecock* in England, and in northern France, the *jeu du Volant*. These games involved using a paddle or a racket to hit an object, probably a piece of cork with some feathers attached, in order to keep it in the air. There are records of similar games all through Asia, so it is not possible to identify a single origin of this type of game. In the 19th century, various English officials learned the game of *Poona* in India. It was very similar to the battledore and shuttlecock of its native England; later on a net was added. Around 1870 the Duke of Beaufort established regulations for play and began organizing matches of this new sport at his country home, Badminton House, the likely source of the name for this discipline.

Tennis player and an engraving of a tennis match, 19th century.

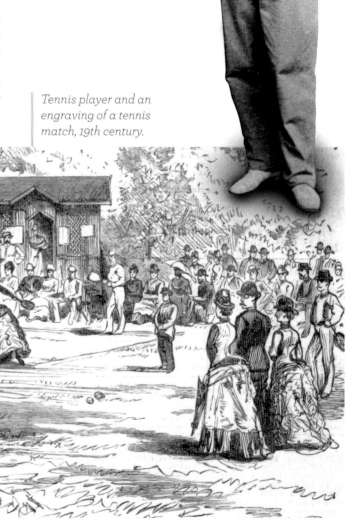

Equipment

In order to play racket or paddle sports we need to use basic equipment that, aside from a few technical qualities, requires no excessive specialization; it merely needs to be adapted to the specific athletic activity that we intend to take up.

CLOTHING

We will begin by describing the basic equipment that all players of racket and paddle sports should use, regardless of which discipline they choose.

Sport or Polo Shirt: It is appropriate to wear a sport or a polo shirt with a breathable weave; it should be comfortable, loose, and lightweight. Cotton garments were used in the past, but nowadays finer, lighter fabrics are used that facilitate sweating and greater cooling of the skin while efficiently wicking away moisture from sweat. This gives the player greater freedom of movement and prevents chafing from constant rubbing in moist areas. For outdoor events clothing of very light colors is recommended that does not absorb the heat from the sun and that keeps the player cool.

Sport Shirt: breathable, with a bit of elasticity; roomy, light in color and weight, permitting total mobility and comforts during extended play, including outdoors.

Shorts: roomy, thin, and breathable to allow total freedom of movement.

Even though it is preferable to wear a loose clothing, many female players choose a tight-fitting tank top with straps and a sports bra for better chest support and greater ease of play in any kind of movement.

Shorts and Skirts: Loose shorts made of light fabrics that do not restrict movement are commonly worn because of the great variety of movements and forced extensions required of the legs in racket and paddle sports. Women also commonly wear skirts with built-in shorts because of the freedom of movement that they provide.

Socks: To a great extent, this article of clothing determines our capacity for play, because of the increased mobility that is required and the long playing times involved in matches. The socks need to be thicker than usual to protect the athlete's feet from continuous rubbing inside the shoe, which results from sudden stops and starts. It's a good idea to choose socks without seams in the areas particularly subject to rubbing, such as the heel and the tips of the toes. There are socks made specifically for players of racket and paddle sports, using reinforced, non-chafing material in these areas, and even elastic thread at the ankle and the middle of the foot to improve the fit and keep the shoe from slipping during play.

Other Items for Safety and Comfort: In situations where profuse sweating is a factor, we can use absorbent elastic headbands to keep the sweat out of our eyes. Sunglasses and brimmed caps will keep the bright sun out of our eyes while playing outdoors. The latter option may limit our field of view slightly, but it will reduce the player's exposure to the sun, so using these items is a personal decision. It is very important to use glasses that were made for playing racket sports, for both the lenses and the frames must be made of tough, shatterproof materials, and they must be constructed so that everything is tough and flexible. In addition to avoiding breakage, this will keep any sharp edges from digging in. Glasses also protect us from getting hit, as with squash goggles.

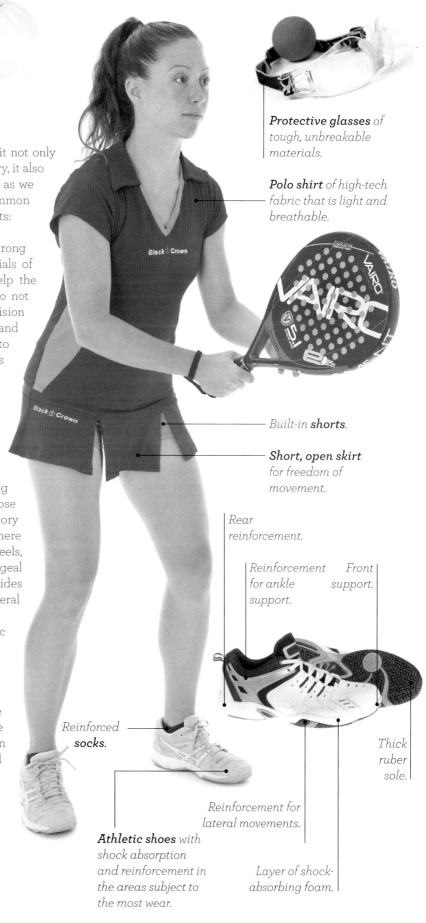

Cap for playing outdoors. It protects the eyes from bright sun and sunstroke. It should be thin, light, and preferably light in color.

FOOTWEAR

This is a very important piece of equipment; it not only protects the feet and ankles from possible injury, it also allows for speedier, more precise play as long as we make the right choice. The following are common features of footwear for racket and paddle sports:

Strength: The shoes must be made of strong materials, whether leather or synthetic materials of similar strength and toughness. This will help the shoes fit your feet snugly so that your feet do not move inside them; this stability will add precision to your movements and protect your ankles and toes. The athletic shoes should be reinforced to support the continuous directional changes involved in play. Shoes that are made of cloth or mesh are good choices.

Traction and Shock Absorption: The sole should be appropriate for the nature of the game; it requires cushioning between the foot and the rubber that contacts the ground, and it should be sufficient for cushioning footfalls. Still, it should not be so thick that you lose precision contact with the ground and satisfactory maneuverability ("feeling the ground"). There should also be reinforcement at the toes, heels, and sides, especially near the metatarsophalangeal joints. The shoes should also be tighter on the sides to provide stability and better grip in the lateral moves that are very common in racket sports.

Finally, the sole needs to have specific shock absorption, traction, and strength characteristics keyed to the playing surface. In general, athletic shoes for clay and grass courts have a lower profile because they need less shock absorption and more control, since we are dealing with surfaces that produce more skidding. The tread pattern is important in determining traction. On hard surfaces (wood floors, cement, asphalt, …), the sole needs to be harder and to provide more shock absorption. The tread is less important because these are surfaces that provide lots of traction.

Protective glasses of tough, unbreakable materials.

Polo shirt of high-tech fabric that is light and breathable.

Built-in shorts.

Short, open skirt for freedom of movement.

Rear reinforcement.

Reinforcement for ankle support.

Front support.

Reinforced socks.

Thick ruber sole.

Reinforcement for lateral movements.

Athletic shoes with shock absorption and reinforcement in the areas subject to the most wear.

Layer of shock-absorbing foam.

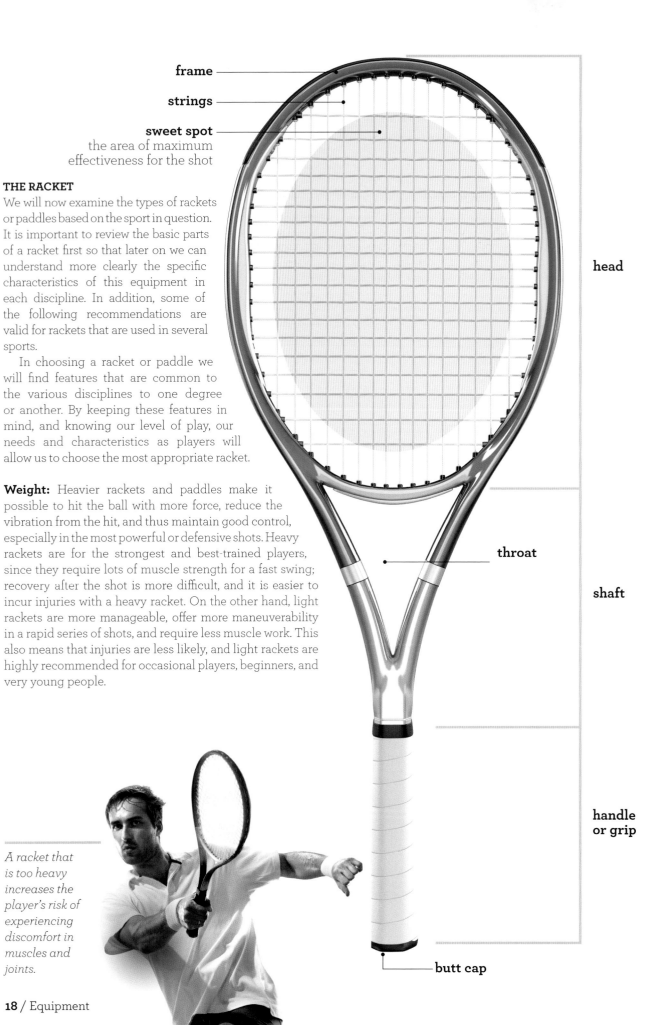

frame

strings

sweet spot
the area of maximum
effectiveness for the shot

head

throat

shaft

handle
or grip

butt cap

THE RACKET

We will now examine the types of rackets or paddles based on the sport in question. It is important to review the basic parts of a racket first so that later on we can understand more clearly the specific characteristics of this equipment in each discipline. In addition, some of the following recommendations are valid for rackets that are used in several sports.

In choosing a racket or paddle we will find features that are common to the various disciplines to one degree or another. By keeping these features in mind, and knowing our level of play, our needs and characteristics as players will allow us to choose the most appropriate racket.

Weight: Heavier rackets and paddles make it possible to hit the ball with more force, reduce the vibration from the hit, and thus maintain good control, especially in the most powerful or defensive shots. Heavy rackets are for the strongest and best-trained players, since they require lots of muscle strength for a fast swing; recovery after the shot is more difficult, and it is easier to incur injuries with a heavy racket. On the other hand, light rackets are more manageable, offer more maneuverability in a rapid series of shots, and require less muscle work. This also means that injuries are less likely, and light rackets are highly recommended for occasional players, beginners, and very young people.

A racket that is too heavy increases the player's risk of experiencing discomfort in muscles and joints.

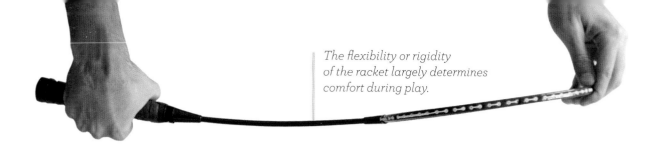

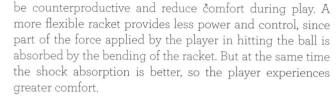

The flexibility or rigidity of the racket largely determines comfort during play.

Length: Long rackets make it possible to apply more force to the shot; they also offer longer reach and a serve at a slightly more advantageous angle. On the other hand, they are less precise and less maneuverable, especially with balls that are headed for your body. Thus, shorter rackets favor maneuverability at the expense of reach and power. The choice depends largely on the player's characteristics. A person with a powerful shot probably will not need to use a long racket and will feel more comfortable with a manageable, flexible one.

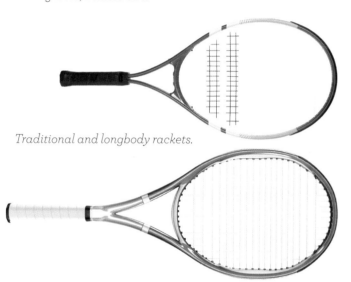

Traditional and longbody rackets.

Balance: The racket's balance point indicates where its center of gravity is located—whether there is more weight toward the head or toward the grip. As we will see, the balance of the racket or paddle can be determined by consulting the specifications that accompany it or by getting help from a professional. Rackets with a center of gravity more toward the head allow for more powerful shots, so they are a good choice for players who need to improve this facet of their game, or whose technique is already advanced. As the center of gravity moves toward the grip, the racket will give up power in the shot, but it will allow greater control, so this type of racket or paddle can be appropriate for players with a very powerful basic shot, or for those whose technical level is not very advanced, such as beginners and casual players who need to focus on control. As their technical level improves, players can use lead-weighted adhesive tape to adjust the balance of their racket.

Stiffness: Rackets with greater rigidity facilitate more powerful shots and greater directional control, but they transmit vibration to the player's hand and wrist, which can be counterproductive and reduce comfort during play. A more flexible racket provides less power and control, since part of the force applied by the player in hitting the ball is absorbed by the bending of the racket. But at the same time the shock absorption is better, so the player experiences greater comfort.

Head Size: This determines the useful striking surface. Rackets with a larger striking surface have a larger "sweet spot," the area that allows hitting the ball and getting a

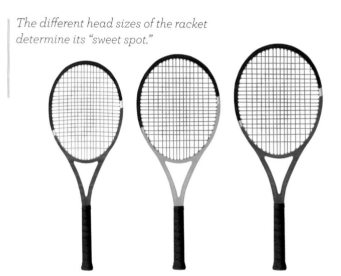

The different head sizes of the racket determine its "sweet spot."

controlled, accurate shot. This type of racket also provides a better launch for the ball, requiring less striking force as long as the ball hits the sweet spot. So these rackets are a good choice for casual and intermediate players. On the other hand, rackets with medium or small areas require a more centered hit, since they offer less leeway; however, at the same time they offer greater directional control.

String Tension: Greater string tension allows better control of the ball, since the shot can be directed with greater precision; but more vibration is transmitted to the arm. On the other hand, lighter string tension will provide a better launch for the ball with less effort, a reduction in directional accuracy, and greater comfort because more vibration is absorbed. In addition, it is possible to use anti-vibration devices; located at the lower part of the strings, they help reduce vibrations from the shot. The most advanced players can choose among different types of strings that vary in thickness, elasticity, and density of string pattern for adaptation to their style of playing.

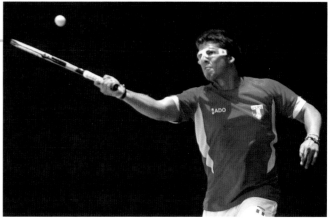

RACKETS, BALLS, AND SHUTTLECOCKS

Badminton: Badminton rackets are characterized by their lightness. They weigh between about 3 and 5¼ ounces (90 and 150 g) when strung. Their light weight and long shaft or spindle make them ideal for a game in which wrist movement is crucially important. Also, this is the only type of racket that allows hitting the shuttlecock with precision. In the interest of lightness, these rackets are designed with a very thin shaft and frame; they are commonly made of aluminum, graphite, or carbon fiber, and the grip is broader for a firm, secure grip. The shuttlecock consists of 16 feathers attached to a half-round base made of cork. These feathers are laced together with thread to give the shuttlecock a conical shape. High-level competition shuttlecocks are often made of natural feathers for better flight and greater precision in hitting. But normally beginner and intermediate players use plastic or nylon shuttlecocks because they are cheaper and last longer.

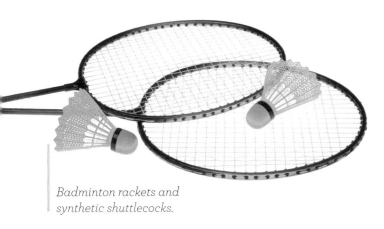

Badminton rackets and synthetic shuttlecocks.

Frontenis: Frontenis rackets generally are quite similar to tennis rackets, and many times tennis rackets are used for playing frontenis with excellent results. Still, it is a good idea to keep a few points in mind for better performance in our playing. First of all, the balls need to have more bounce, since very long or very powerful shots are needed to reach the front wall from the back of the court and produce sufficient bounce; thus it is important to choose a racket with characteristics that facilitate powerful shots, even though this involves a certain loss of precision. For example, the racket can be heavier, have a broad hitting area, or be long. The ball is rubber with no covering; generally it is yellow or blue, and it is smaller and has greater bounce than a tennis ball.

Paddleball: Based on the materials inside, we distinguish between EVA (ethylene-vinyl acetate) rubber and ones made of polyurethane foam. The former material is harder, so it behaves similar to a tightly strung racket, but with better vibration absorption and tolerance of powerful shots. Foam is softer, and it is like a tightly strung racket, which gives it a more resilient shot and better vibration absorption than EVA rubber. The surface of the paddle may be either smooth or rough. The latter aids in emphasizing the effects imparted to the ball, due to greater adherence in topspin shots.

Another feature to keep in mind is balance. In the most rudimentary paddles, the shape of the head can be an indicator. Because of the distribution of the material, diamond-shaped paddles tend to have a high balance point, in other words, toward the end of the head. This increases power at the expense of control, and makes them more

diamond	teardrop	round

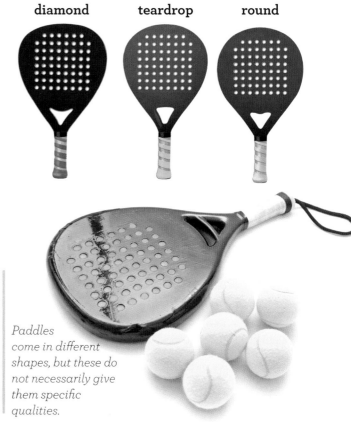

Paddles come in different shapes, but these do not necessarily give them specific qualities.

appropriate for advanced players. The opposite is the case with round heads, and the center of gravity is closer to the grip, which provides greater control and less power. In the middle we find paddles with a teardrop shape, with a greater balance between the two types.

We have to remember that nowadays, especially in medium and top-of-the-line paddles, the manufacturers can alter densities and amounts of materials, along with weight distribution, to adapt them to different playing styles, so oftentimes the shape of the paddles does not determine its qualities and we will need to get help from a specialist to make the right choice.

The balls used in paddleball are very similar to tennis balls, and their most noteworthy variation is that they are lower in pressure; this produces a shorter bounce and facilitates play in a smaller space.

Squash: Materials keep getting lighter and tougher, such as aluminum, graphite, titanium, and carbon fiber, which are used to make rackets that weigh no more than 4¼ ounces (120 g) when strung. We should keep in mind the narrowness of the shaft, since even though a thinner shaft affords greater maneuverability of the racket, a thicker one makes for more powerful shots. Here too we need to consider the balance of the racket and make our choice based on our level and style of playing. This is not so easy to determine from the shape

of the head, but it will be part of the product specifications. The thinner and longer shape of the racket favors the wrist movement necessary for hitting a light ball like the one used in squash. The ball is smaller in size, black, and very low-pressure to reduce the bounce and to speed up the game. In competition, a ball with two yellow dots is used; this is the best choice for advanced players. A ball with just one yellow dot is similar to the previous one, but it has more bounce, which increases the hang time and makes for slightly slower play. A ball with a red dot is a bit larger and has more bounce than the previous one, so the game is slower; this is a good choice for occasional players. Finally, a ball with a blue dot is larger and slower, and is the ideal choice for beginners.

Tennis: All the general guidelines relative to length, weight, stiffness, head size, and string tension already mentioned are applicable to tennis rackets. The balance point is often in the neck of the racket: the acronym HH means *heavy head*, and LH, *light head*. In the former, the center of gravity is closer to the head, and in the latter, closer to the handle. These letters are often accompanied with the number of inches. The larger this number, the more noticeable the displacement of the center of gravity toward the head or the grip, and this has ramifications for every player. Finally, the balls are made of rubber; they weigh two ounces (58 g), and are covered with felt, which dampens the bounce and the hit, as well as reduce their speed.

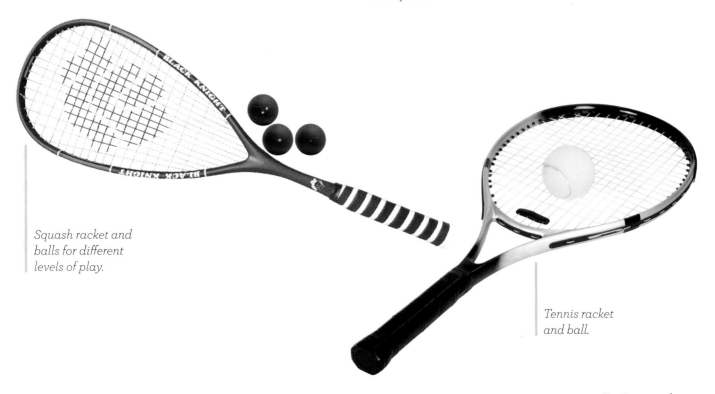

Squash racket and balls for different levels of play.

Tennis racket and ball.

Shots and Biomechanics

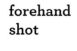

forehand shot

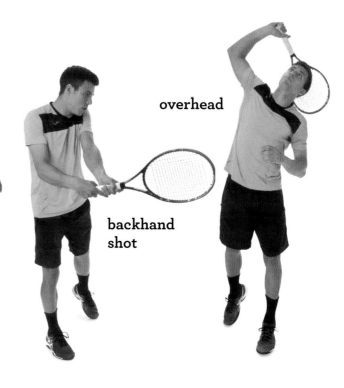

overhead

backhand shot

In this section we will address the basic, common shots that we encounter in racket and paddle sports, their physical requirements, and their main biomechanical characteristics. People who are familiar with the racket sports know that there is a broad variety of shots and that every one of them can entail many variants. It would be a huge task to do a detailed study of all of them.

In this instance, we will restrict ourselves to the forehand, the backhand, and the overhead, since these are the three that epitomize the main variations in physical requirements for the upper body and limbs; we will skip over the running requirements for the lower body, since they are covered in many other publications.

By knowing these shots we can identify where the effort is concentrated in the performance of each one of them, and we will be able to do the right physical training for the best performance in the game. In addition, with this knowledge and everything we have learned about equipment and injuries, which we will address in the next section, we can act to prevent any symptom of strain and possible injury, thereby protecting our physical well-being.

We should remember that in general the contraction of a muscle causes a stretch in its antagonist, and in racket and paddle sports, where most shots make use of a certain elastic component that is favored by the sequence of backswing-acceleration-shot, it is important to work not only the muscles that actively contract during the performance of the technical movement, but also the ones that stretch in the preparation or the execution, are used in braking the momentum from the hit, or experience a quick succession of extension and contraction.

We should point out that the practice of any racket or paddle sport tends to cause asymmetry in the player's muscles and tendons. This is most noticeable in the upper extremities, present in the torso, and less significant or absent in the lower limbs, as a result of the dominant side that is used to manipulate the racket. It is easy to see this asymmetry in some players at very high levels, such as Rafa Nadal, whose left arm is much more muscular than his right, since he is left-handed. So it is clear that the first recommendation for maintaining the optimal, balanced athlete who does not aspire to join the ranks of the elite is to do compensating exercises to strengthen the non-dominant side, and to increase flexibility and encourage recuperation in the dominant one.

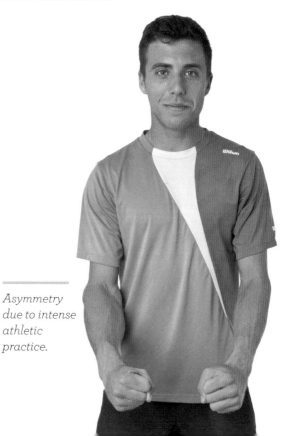

Asymmetry due to intense athletic practice.

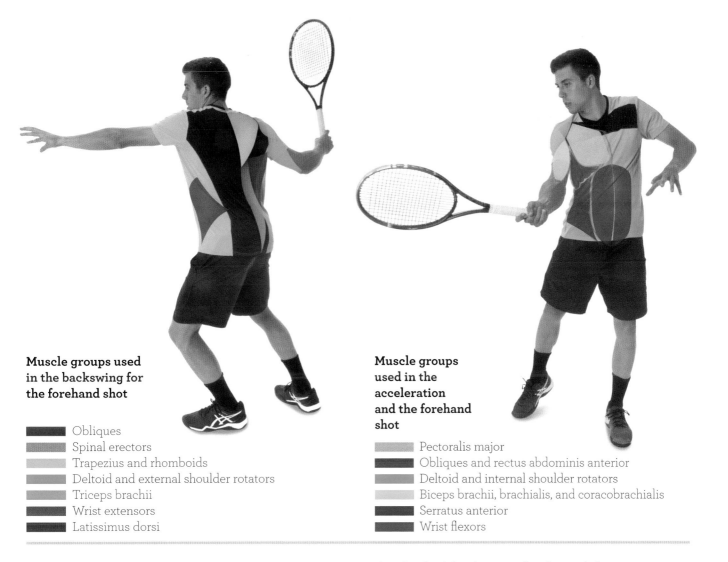

Muscle groups used in the backswing for the forehand shot

- ▬ Obliques
- ▬ Spinal erectors
- ▬ Trapezius and rhomboids
- ▬ Deltoid and external shoulder rotators
- ▬ Triceps brachii
- ▬ Wrist extensors
- ▬ Latissimus dorsi

Muscle groups used in the acceleration and the forehand shot

- ▬ Pectoralis major
- ▬ Obliques and rectus abdominis anterior
- ▬ Deltoid and internal shoulder rotators
- ▬ Biceps brachii, brachialis, and coracobrachialis
- ▬ Serratus anterior
- ▬ Wrist flexors

THE FOREHAND SHOT

This shot is the one used most frequently in a match, so in addition to the physical requirements of the shot itself there is the necessity of repeating it hundreds of times throughout a match and in training sessions. This is also the shot that produces the greatest precision and accuracy with the ball, and it can be used both defensively and offensively. We will point to three fundamental phases that are basic to the biomechanical analysis, even though there are more detailed breakdowns, mainly for analyzing them technically.

Backswing: In this phase of the movement the dominant arm and the racket move rearward with respect to the body in order to gain space for the acceleration of the following phase and take advantage of the elastic component. First of all, it is necessary to rotate and extend the upper body by using the abdominal muscles, mainly the internal and external obliques, plus the spinal erectors, especially in the lumbar area. This first upper-body rotation will be accompanied by a horizontal abduction of the shoulder and a scapular adduction, as well as a partial extension of the elbow and the wrist in the dominant arm. This movement will involve mainly the trapezius, greater and lesser rhomboids, deltoid, triceps brachii, and the wrist extensor muscles, although we should not overlook the involvement of other muscles such as the external shoulder rotators and the latissimus dorsi.

Acceleration and Shot: This phase of the movement is more exacting than the previous one, since it requires greater power and is the main one used in the shot. It follows a direction opposite that of the backswing, using an elastic, explosive movement that creates forward acceleration of the racket to hit the ball efficiently. The upper body will need to rotate in the direction opposite the backswing, like a slight flex in which the internal obliques, external obliques, and rectus abdominis are used. The movement of the shoulder, elbow, and wrist will involve the pectoralis major, the deltoid, the biceps brachii, the brachioradialis, and the wrist flexor muscles, plus the internal shoulder rotators and the serratus anterior.

Follow-through: The swing of the racket continues after it connects with the ball. The swing continues upward, and it emphasizes the simultaneous flex in the elbow and wrist. Repetition of this movement is the cause of epitrochleitis or "golfer's elbow."

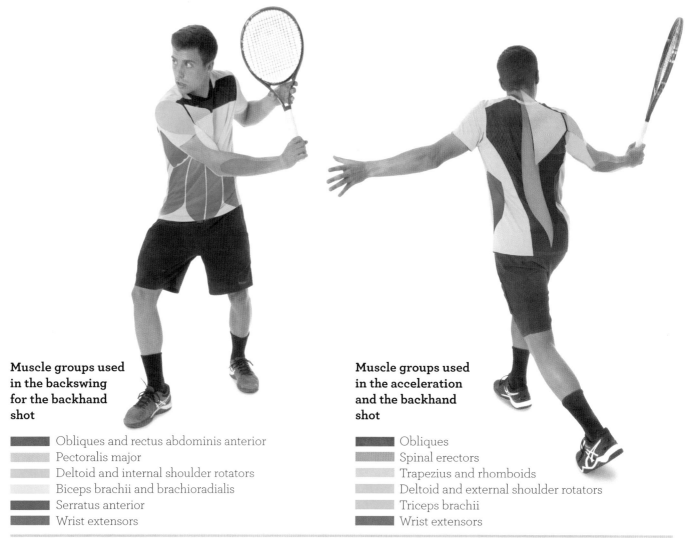

Muscle groups used in the backswing for the backhand shot

▬ Obliques and rectus abdominis anterior
▬ Pectoralis major
▬ Deltoid and internal shoulder rotators
▬ Biceps brachii and brachioradialis
▬ Serratus anterior
▬ Wrist extensors

Muscle groups used in the acceleration and the backhand shot

▬ Obliques
▬ Spinal erectors
▬ Trapezius and rhomboids
▬ Deltoid and external shoulder rotators
▬ Triceps brachii
▬ Wrist extensors

THE BACKHAND SHOT

This shot is less common than the forehand, but it is still used very frequently and it requires intensive use of the muscles that rotate the upper body and the one that originates at the lateral epicondyle of the humerus. There is a reason why this shot is the main one that causes lumbar pain that many players experience, and epicondylitis or "tennis elbow." When two hands are used for the backhand, the upper-body muscles are the ones that bear the greatest burden; in a one-handed backhand most of the load falls on the dominant arm and shoulder.

Backswing: The player must move the dominant arm and the racket rearward as in the forehand shot, but this time the arm will cross in front of the body via rotation of the torso and horizontal shoulder adduction. The internal obliques, external obliques, and the rectus abdominis play a major role in this upper-body movement and setup. As in the previous case, the racket is brought far back in anticipation of the acceleration. The pectoralis major, deltoid, biceps brachii, brachioradialis, wrist flexor muscles, internal shoulder rotators, and serratus anterior are particularly important in the movement of the shoulder and the arm.

Shot: In the backhand this phase likewise produces the acceleration by reversing the backswing movement, applying greater force to transmit power to the ball. This phase involves activating the upper-body extensor muscles, especially in the lumbar area, as well as the major and minor obliques to produce the rotation, which needs to be much more pronounced and rapid in the two-handed backhand to compensate for the limited mobility resulting from the two-handed grip.

The arm movement will require the use of the trapezius, major and minor rhomboids, deltoid, triceps brachii, and the wrist extensors, plus the latissimus dorsi and the external shoulder rotators.

In this movement, the simultaneous extension of the wrist and elbow seems to be the main cause of epicondylitis.

Follow-through: As with the previous case, the movement does not stop abruptly, and the horizontal shoulder abduction is continued, along with the wrist extension. However, the elbow regains a certain degree of bend before the movement stops entirely.

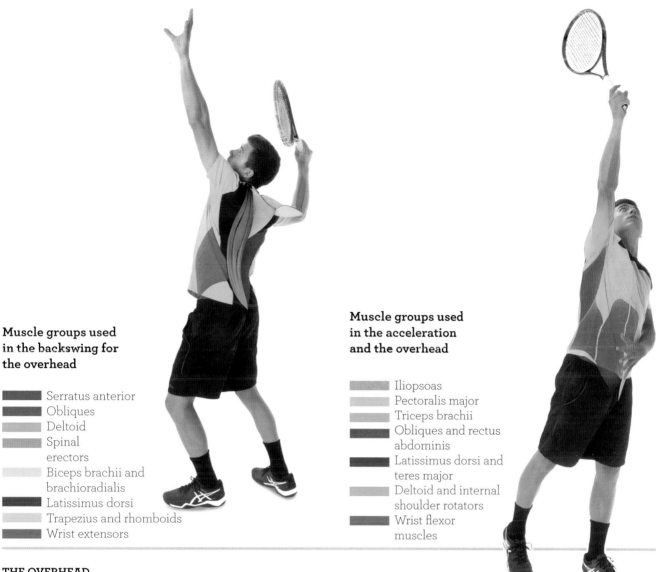

Muscle groups used in the backswing for the overhead

- Serratus anterior
- Obliques
- Deltoid
- Spinal erectors
- Biceps brachii and brachioradialis
- Latissimus dorsi
- Trapezius and rhomboids
- Wrist extensors

Muscle groups used in the acceleration and the overhead

- Iliopsoas
- Pectoralis major
- Triceps brachii
- Obliques and rectus abdominis
- Latissimus dorsi and teres major
- Deltoid and internal shoulder rotators
- Wrist flexor muscles

THE OVERHEAD

This shot clearly is a powerful, offensive one that follows a sharply downward trajectory. It probably also makes greater use of the elastic component of the oblique anterior muscle chain, and is more dangerous for the abdominal muscles and the hip flexor, precisely because of the sudden change involved in the extension and contraction of the upper body, which is the source for some of the power that is transmitted to the ball and makes it almost impossible to reach. We must keep in mind that this movement is less common in squash and more highly valued in tennis, where the serve retains great similarity to the overhead on a biomechanical level, and in badminton.

Backswing: In this phase of the overhead the idea is to arch the body to create the greatest elastic component and the longest route for the acceleration. This requires the basic components of maximum extension and a slight upper-body rotation. We must remember the bend in the shoulder and elbow of the playing arm, which will complete the shape of an arc. The spinal erectors and the internal and external obliques are involved in the extension and rotation of the upper body. The deltoid, biceps brachii, brachioradialis, serratus anterior, and the wrist extensors are used in the movement of the shoulder and arm.

Shot: We make use of the elastic component of the abdominal muscles and the hip flexor, as well as the shoulder extensor muscles. The upper body flexes very quickly, along with the hip, though to a lesser degree in the latter case, by reversing the arc and providing a certain amount of acceleration. To this is added the extension of the shoulder and elbow, plus the bend in the hip, which acts like a catapult or a trebuchet to create the maximum acceleration in the racket, and thus an extremely powerful shot. In ascending anatomical order, the muscles involved are the iliopsoas muscles, the internal and external obliques, the rectus abdominis, and in the mobilization of the shoulder and arm, the latissimus dorsi, teres major, pectoralis major, deltoid, triceps brachii, wrist flexors, and internal shoulder rotators.

Follow-through: The motion must continue after the ball is hit; this makes for a more fluid motion and allows the racket and arm to brake more gradually, particularly in a shot like this one, where the ball can reach very high speed.

Injuries

In this section we will briefly present some of the injuries that afflict players of racket and paddle sports, along with the mechanisms that cause them. Prior conditioning and muscle flexibility may help prevent most of them.

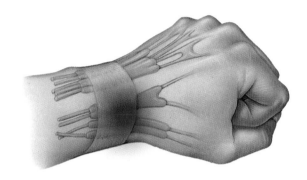

De Quervain's tenosynovitis causes wrist pain near the base of the thumb.

De Quervain's Tenosynovitis: This discomfort affects the tendons of the adductor longus and the extensor brevis of the thumb. These tendons are covered by a synovial membrane that allows them to slide inside the sheath that covers them. Intensive use of the adductor longus muscle and the extensor brevis pollicis and/or the opposing muscles, plus the repetitive movement of the wrist, especially the abduction-adduction sequence, can produce inflammation of the tendons and enlargement of the whole structure, causing pain in the wrist at the base of the thumb. Because of the continual gripping and use of the racket or paddle during a game, athletes in these specialties are more prone to experiencing this complaint, so it is a good idea to do stretching exercises for the area involved.

Tendonitis in the Wrist Flexors and Extensors: Wrist flexion and extension are movements that are repeated many times during play, and the muscles involved have to overcome resistance from the weight of the racket and absorb the vibrations generated by the impact of the ball against it. This can affect the tendons at the distal insertion of the wrist flexor and extensor muscles and even cause them to become inflamed, with attendant pain. Forehand shots, overheads, and serves in tennis affect the anterior part of the wrist, and backhands have a greater effect on the posterior part. Thus, it is a good idea to do strengthening work and stretches for this musculature at the end of an athletic training session.

Epicondylitis or "Tennis Elbow": This affects the tendons that insert into the epicondyle of the wrist extensor muscles. During the backhand shot the effect is extension of the wrist and supination of the forearm, with the application of considerable force and subsequent absorption of the impact from the ball. The repetition of this motion, especially against resistance, is the main cause for this complaint, although excessive elbow extension during the shot, a change of racket, the strings, and their tension may also be triggers. This problem is common in players who practice regularly, and with lesser frequency in experienced players; it is accompanied by pain in the outer side of the elbow. Besides strengthening and stretching the wrist extensor muscles, this discomfort can be prevented by using a proper grip, moving the shot forward so that the racket hits the ball in front of the body, or making greater use of the two-handed backhand shot, which reduces the effort in the wrist.

Epicondylitis or tennis elbow is common among players of racket sports.

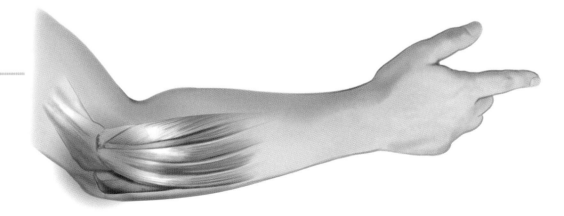

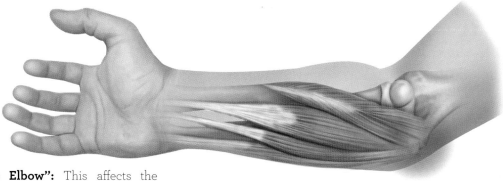

Epitrochleitis or "Golfer's Elbow": This affects the tendons that insert at the epitrochlea of the wrist flexor muscles. Even though those who play racket and paddle sports are not the ones most affected by this ailment (as the name indicates), we need to point out that repeated flexing of the wrist and pronation of the forearm, especially against resistance, are the main drivers of epitrochleitis. This motion is repeated in the forehand shot, especially with topspin, and in the overhead or tennis serve, so this is a fairly common ailment that affects experienced players in particular who spend many hours in practice. It shows up as pain in the inside face of the elbow, and stretches for the epitrochlear muscles; strengthening them with specific exercises can help with prevention.

Pain at the Rear of the Elbow: This is often due to the repetitive use of the backhand shot with complete extension of the elbow. This action, with an abrupt end to the motion and maximum elbow extension, can produce an impact between the olecranon and the olecranal fossa and produce pain in the posterior part of the elbow. We recommend eliminating the abrupt ending of the motion and shortening it slightly if possible. Also, by way of prevention, it is important to do strengthening work for the elbow flexor muscles and for flexibility in the extensors.

Tendonitis of the Biceps Brachii: This is the result of repeated shots that require simultaneous flexion of the elbow and shoulder, as in the forehand shot, especially with topspin, and to a greater degree with a higher ending of the motion. It affects the origin of the large head of the biceps brachii, and it commonly appears as pain in the anterior face of the shoulder. Strengthening exercises for the biceps brachii contribute to prevention.

Inflammation of the Rotator Cuff: Discomfort in the shoulders regularly or occasionally affects a third of young players and half of veterans. It may result from insufficient conditioning and preparation of the shoulder rotator muscles, whose tendons can become inflamed through excessive use and cause inflammation of the sac that covers them, but in most instances it is due to repetitive high shots, such as overheads and serves in tennis, which require bending the shoulder above 90°. Above this angle, it is common for the sac for the rotators to get pinched between the humerus and the acromion. If this process is repeated, it can result in inflammation of the tendons or the sac (bursa) that facilitates their sliding, and this causes pain in the shoulder. Strengthening the rotator muscles involved and limiting the movements that raise the arm higher than shoulder level can be effective prevention measures.

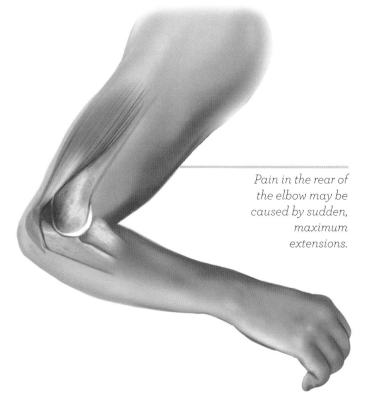

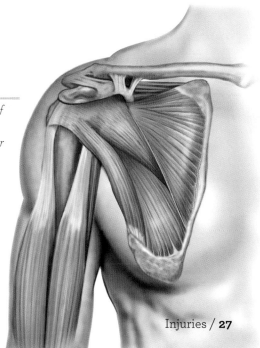

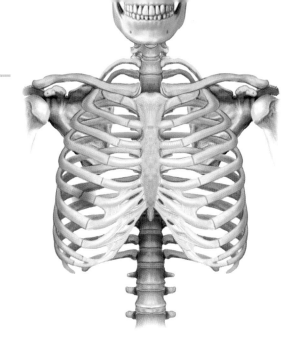

SLAP-type Injuries: This name is an acronym for *Superior Labrum from Anterior to Posterior*. This injury affects the glenoid labrum, which is a stabilizing element in the shoulder. The injury is produced by maximum horizontal abduction movements of the shoulder, like the ones that are done between the backswing and the acceleration for the forehand shot. It also affects baseball pitchers and handball players, since the movements are similar. Extreme ranges of movement and abrupt execution are commonly the sources of this injury, but there may also be a degenerative cause, and it can affect both young and veteran players. When this injury appears, it requires surgical repair. It manifests as pain in the shoulder, and depending on degree, it causes greater or lesser instability in the joint, so repeated dislocations may result if athletic activity is not stopped.

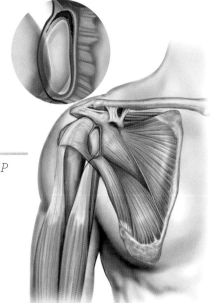

An injury of the SLAP type is relatively common in athletes who perform abrupt movements with the shoulder during play.

Rib Fracture or Fissure Due to Stress or Strain: This is not very common, but it can happen through intense, repeated traction of some muscles that originate or insert at the ribs, for example the obliques and the serratus anterior, which are used intensively in various moves in racket sports. This injury can range from discomfort while coughing, laughing, or breathing deeply, to thoracic pain. It can be prevented with adequate physical conditioning and flexibility work for the muscles involved. Stress and overload fractures can occur in other areas of the body as a result of the repeated tension that some powerful muscles can exert on bones, and the impacts that they experience,

for example while running. It is not uncommon for stress or strain fractures to appear on the tibia and the fibula; they can be prevented with stretching exercises and the wearing of shoes that dampen the impact from running.

Abdominal and Groin Injuries: Muscular injuries in these areas are common in racket and paddle sports. This is due to making shots such as the overhead and the serve in tennis, which require stretching of the abdominal and the hip flexor muscles during the backswing, and then their sudden contraction during the acceleration and the shot. The upper-body rotation involves not only the rectus abdominis, but also the oblique muscles, so it is important to strengthen the abdominal wall and provide it with enough flexibility to absorb the forces of stretching and contraction that act on it. This type of injury appears as pain in the abdominal wall or the groin, and it is more common among athletes whose disciplines involve more high shots, as with badminton players.

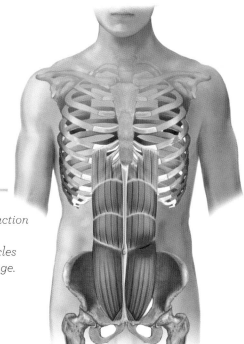

An abrupt extension-contraction sequence of the abdominal muscles can cause damage.

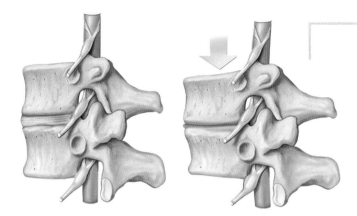

The forces of compression, torsion, and shearing that act on intervertebral discs can cause pain, especially in the lumbar area.

Rupture of the Medial Head of the Gastrocnemius, or "Tennis Leg": This muscle rupture, whether partial or total, arises from the repeated abrupt running starts when, for example, the player has to reach a short shot or a let ball. It is not very common in very young players, but it can affect them too if their physical preparation is poor, because of the demands that the racket sports place on the lower body. It affects mainly players older than 35, who should pay particular attention to strength and flexibility work for the gastrocnemius muscles as a way to prevent this injury. "Tennis leg" produces intense pain along with a click upon starting to run that has been likened to getting hit with a rock. Edema may appear, plus, depending on the seriousness of the injury, pain while walking and even total functional inability to walk.

Back Pain: Even though this is not strictly an injury, it can be an indicator or a harbinger of future injuries. It can appear in the flexions, extensions, and rotations of the upper body that occur during play, especially if they are abrupt. Shots such as a tennis serve, overhead, or backhand, especially with two hands, are some of the factors that can cause the appearance of back pain. This is due to the forces of compression, torsion, and shearing that act on the intervertebral discs while performing these shots. The pain commonly appears in the lumbar spine, and even though it is more common among veterans, it can also appear in the youngest players. As a preventive measure it is important to strengthen the lumbar and abdominal muscles to provide stability and protection to the area, paying particular attention to compensating exercises.

Knee Pain: As with the previous case, this pain is not an injury, but it may indicate an imbalance that will turn into an injury, or it may indicate an existing injury. Some common injuries are tendonitis of the quadriceps or the kneecap, which are associated with pain in the front of the knee, above or below the kneecap, respectively. Other less common problems are tendonitis of the pes anserinus (goosefoot), of the iliotibial band, and of the biceps femoris, which appear as pain on the inside, the outside, and the posterior face of the knee, respectively. All these discomforts are associated with the running involved in racket sports and others, and players can take preventive measures such as strength work and stretching the muscles that activate the knee. In racket and paddle sports there is one determining factor in their appearance: the abruptness used in successive starts, stops, and changes of direction.

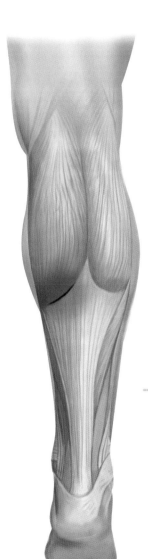

"Tennis leg" is a muscle injury that commonly affects middle-aged players.

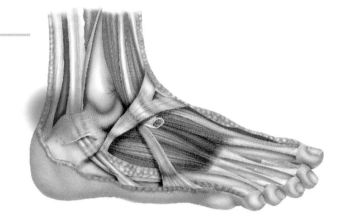

Pain in the rear of the ankle is a warning sign for tendonitis of the Achilles tendon.

Tendonitis of the Achilles Tendon: This can occur in all players who run short distances at high speed; for example, in running to reach a ball, especially if they are very fast or aggressive, like some squash players. Jumps, which also involve plantar flexion of the ankle, may also favor the incidence of this ailment, which appears as pain in the rear of the ankle. It can be prevented with stretching exercises for the gastrocnemius and the soleus, and by avoiding the use of very flat footwear.

Tendonitis of the Tibialis Posterior: This injury is caused similarly to tendonitis of the Achilles tendon; basically, it is due to repeated plantar flexion of the ankle while running. Recommendations for prevention are the same as for tendonitis of the Achilles tendon, since this type of work can prevent both injuries.

Tibial Periostitis: Also known as Medial Tibial Stress Syndrome (MTSS) and shin splints, this ailment is the result of the repeated impact involved in running, especially if we use footwear with inadequate cushioning or play on hard surfaces such as cement or asphalt, which are commonly encountered in frontenis and tennis. It appears as pain in the anterior face of the leg, and stretching exercises for the muscles used in dorsal ankle flexion may help with prevention.

Pereoneal Tendonitis: This appears as pain in the outer face of the ankle, and it is common in racket sports due to the high incidence of lateral movements. Movements through the back of the court or at the net are done in this way, requiring eversion of the ankle with every step, and consequently work from the peroneus muscles that far exceeds the requirements of daily life or other sports that likewise involve running. Even though this is not one of the most common problems among players in these disciplines, we should be aware of it, and players should regularly do exercises for keeping the peroneus muscles flexible and strengthening them.

Ankle Sprain: This generally results from a twist; it is more common in racket sports than in other disciplines, due to the continual running to the side and the attendant eversion and inversion motions of the ankle. These contacts in a position that is unlike what we experience while walking or running straight ahead entail a reduction in the equilibrium of the ankle and a greater risk of twisting and a resultant sprain. This injury is more common in net sports that involve greater movement to the side or to the back of the court. It is important to strengthen the muscles responsible for ankle inversion and eversion, and to do exercises on movable surfaces in the gym (bosu ballast ball) as a means of prevention, and for improvement in the ability to react to being off-balance.

Tibial periostitis (shin splints) is fairly common in runners.

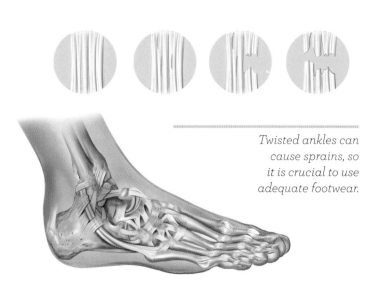

Twisted ankles can cause sprains, so it is crucial to use adequate footwear.

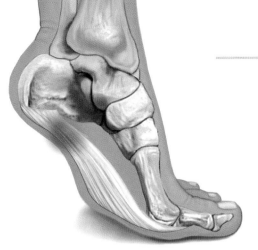

*Stretching the toes
and the sole of the
foot helps prevent
plantar fasciitis.*

require very powerful movements are more susceptible. This happens in racket and paddle sports, since they require power in making shots and in running. To prevent these injuries, it is important to keep the muscles in the best possible condition for strength and flexibility, but above all, a proper, sufficient warm-up before starting intense athletic practice is necessary.

Sprains and Muscle and Tendon Ruptures: In most instances, these injuries occur due to the same forces that cause muscle strains and pulls, and they are more common in disciplines that require sudden, quick, and powerful movements and shifts. So it is natural to think that disciplines such as squash may be particularly affected, given the tremendous speed of play. We must keep in mind that very hard or sticky surfaces allow for less reaction time and no sliding, so athletes who play on this type of court will be more exposed to possible injuries.

Plantar Fasciitis: This is an inflammation of the plantar aponeurosis (fascia), a membrane of connective tissue that runs from the heel to the base of the toes. This membrane gives support to the plantar arch and is subjected to great tension during running. So all athletes whose disciplines involve running are prone to experience plantar fasciitis, including people who play racket sports, and especially those who run longer distances or frequently. This ailment can be prevented with stretches for the plantar fascia and the muscles that perform plantar ankle flexion, plus the proper footwear. There are other types of discomfort that may affect the muscles in the sole of the foot, and their origin is the same as for plantar fasciitis. In these instances, the stretches indicated for the plantar fascia and work to strengthen the muscles will help with prevention.

Muscle Pull and Strain: This condition appears when a muscle exceeds its elastic limit and there is a plastic deformation in the tissue; in other words, there is so much tension that the muscle is unable to return to its original state. This is not limited to a specific muscle or athletic discipline, and it can occur in any muscle that is subjected to forces and sudden tension. Athletes whose disciplines

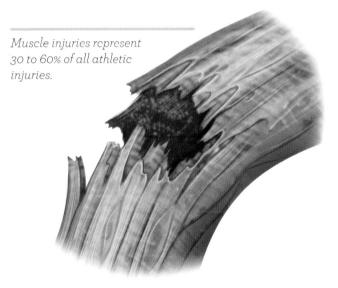

*Muscle injuries represent
30 to 60% of all athletic
injuries.*

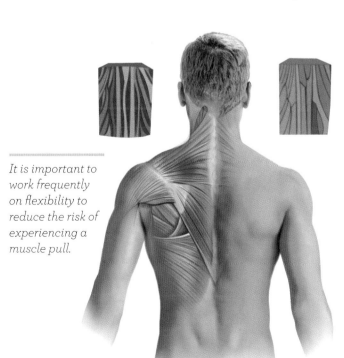

*It is important to
work frequently
on flexibility to
reduce the risk of
experiencing a
muscle pull.*

In this section we have not presented all the injuries that may result from trauma—and there are many—mainly because we have already provided information about proper equipment for preventing trauma from the impact of the ball with serious consequences, and because the other traumas, such as the ones that result from a fall, do not exhibit specific characteristics or differences with respect to the ones that can occur in other sports.

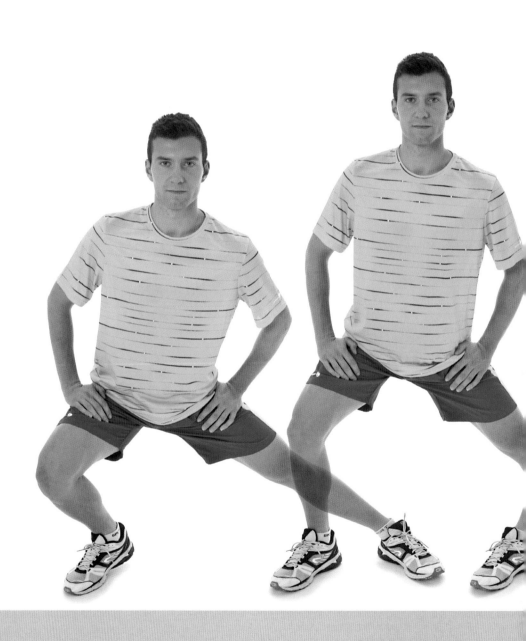

DYNAMIC
STRETCHES

THE BASICS OF DYNAMIC STRETCHES

Dynamic stretches are still great unknowns to many trainers, coaches, and sports professionals. For many years they have dealt with ballistic stretches and the attendant risk of injury, so they have been cast aside and are now used only in some spheres of professional sports, such as sprinting, throwing events, and martial arts, which requires great range of movement combined with powerful moves.

However, the most recent studies seem to indicate that dynamic stretches offer many advantages over static ones at certain times, or if specific results are sought. Dynamic stretches make it possible to achieve a good range of motion in the joints involved, without harming power or explosiveness, so they can help improve performance at the same time that the muscle activity contributes to the warm-up.

Until a short time ago, it was the general belief that including static stretches in the warm-up routine brought many beneficial effects, such as better performance, reduced probability of injury, and even a reduction in recovery time for muscle pain after exercise. Trainers, coaches, and even physical education teachers and professors considered these benefits to be a given, and even today most athletes use static stretches during their warm-ups prior to athletic or competitive activity.

With the most recent scientific data in hand, everything seems to indicate that static stretching before athletic practice does not reduce the risk of injury, and what's worse, it in fact significantly reduces the power, speed, potency, and precision of the movements—all of which are essential for racket sports.

Various high-jumping trials have revealed that individuals who did static stretching before jumping performed below the level of those who did not stretch, and far below those who did a dynamic warm-up routine.

Also, the warm-up is an essential factor for any athlete, especially for those whose discipline requires speed, power, or maximum strength. The warm-up greatly improves the subsequent performance, and it has been clearly proven that it reduces the risk of injuries during athletic activity.

We can conclude that static stretching prior to athletic activity contributes nothing to players of tennis, paddleball, squash, badminton, and other similar sports where the shots and running generally require power and great precision, and that a warm-up that includes dynamism and movement makes it possible to raise the muscle temperature and improve irrigation and oxygenation to the muscles—certainly appropriate preparation for

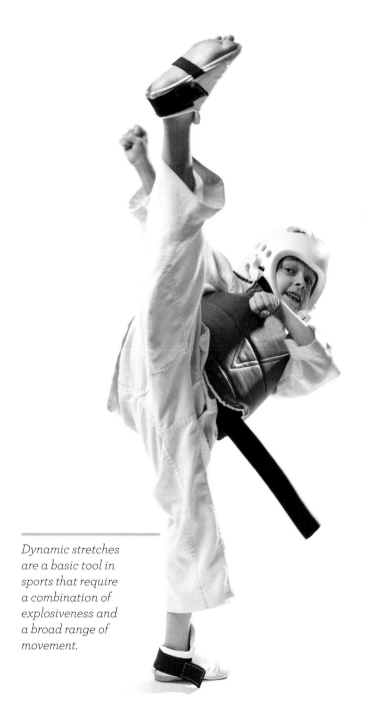

Dynamic stretches are a basic tool in sports that require a combination of explosiveness and a broad range of movement.

competing or doing a hard workout with the best assurances for performance and health.

If we analyze dynamic stretches thoroughly, we see that they contain some promising elements for people who play racket and paddle sports, because of the special characteristics they have and the explosiveness that they require in many of the movements.

The circumduction of the shoulders that tennis players, baseball pitchers, handball players, and others often perform before a game is nothing more than a dynamic way to perform a broad movement in the shoulder joint to prepare that joint and the muscles that operate it for the intense activity that will follow.

So the benefits of dynamic stretches prior to playing a sport are clear. Now we should focus on some guidelines on how to do them to get the maximum benefit and avoid possible injuries connected to improper execution:

■ Dynamic stretching should be understood as a series of connected stretches—a cycle of movements that is repeated in succession and without pause for a desired period of time.

■ The movement used in stretching a muscle group should entail a certain level of momentum or speed, but without becoming abrupt or uncontrolled at any time, since this would involve a risk to the joints, tendons, muscles, and ligaments.

■ At the end of the movement used for the stretch there should be a small bounce to help reach the range of motion necessary for improved flexibility.

■ The duration of a set will be applied to all movement cycles, not to a static position.

Finally, it is important to remember that dynamic stretches should be part of a complete warm-up that should include, among other things, a gentle run that can include some of the chosen stretches.

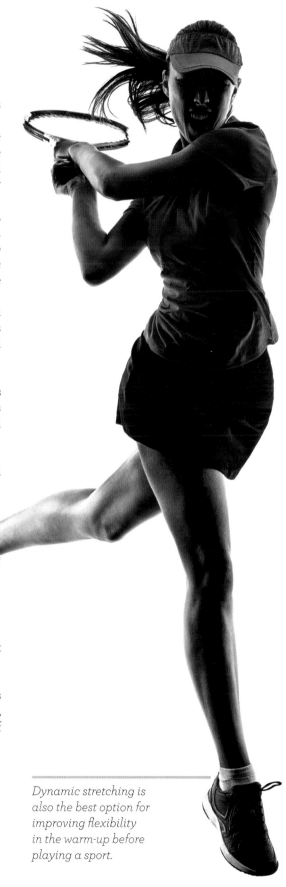

Dynamic stretching is also the best option for improving flexibility in the warm-up before playing a sport.

Bilateral Windmill

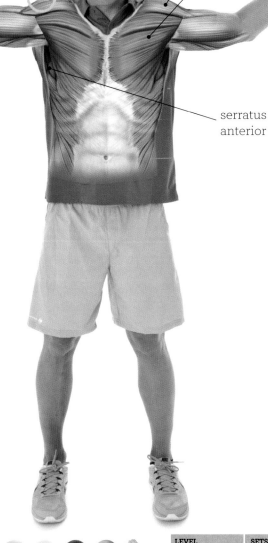

Keep your back straight.

deltoid

pectoralis major

serratus anterior

START
Stand with your feet about shoulder width apart. Your arms should hang loose at your sides, with your elbows straight and your forearms and hands in relaxed, natural pronation.

TECHNIQUE
Raise your arms toward the front using shoulder flexion, as you simultaneously bend your elbows slightly. Continue raising and separating your hands and keep them moving so that both arms describe a circular movement toward the rear and downward. When they reach the bottom, keep them moving and repeat the cycle. This circumduction with both arms can be done in either direction, and you can even change back and forth in the same set.

Movement Sequence

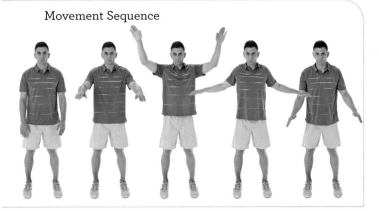

TENNIS	PADDLE.	SQUASH	FRONT.	BADMIN.
✔	✔	✔	✔	✔

LEVEL	SETS	DURATION
BEGINNER	2	30 s
INTERMEDIATE	3	30 s
ADVANCED	3	30 s

CAUTION
You should use some momentum in the movement, but without being too quick or uncontrolled, since excessive speed and sudden bounces are potentially dangerous in dynamic and ballistic stretches. If you feel any grinding in your shoulder, reduce the maximum height of the movement so that your elbows scarcely go higher than shoulder level.

INDICATION
For athletes in racket or paddle sports because of the special involvement of the shoulder joint and the muscles that operate it in the various shots. This exercise helps relieve strain and tension, as well as improve range of motion, which makes for a more fluid and efficient shot.

Alternate Arm Movement

teres major

deltoid

pectoralis major

latissimus dorsi

serratus anterior

coraco-brachialis

biceps brachii

Keep your upper body and legs in line.

START
Standing with your feet separated, raise one arm as high as possible using shoulder flexion. The other shoulder can remain in maximum extension, with one hand high and the other one low as you make crossing arcs with both of them.

TECHNIQUE
Raise the shoulder in flexion as high as possible while the extended shoulder performs the opposite movement, such that both arms coincide at the midpoint of their trajectory. At this point do the movement in the opposite direction and continue the cycle the appropriate number of times.

	TENNIS	PADDLE.	SQUASH	FRONT.	BADMIN.
	✔			✔	✔

LEVEL	SETS	DURATION
BEGINNER	2	20 s
INTERMEDIATE	2	25 s
ADVANCED	3	25 s

Movement Sequence

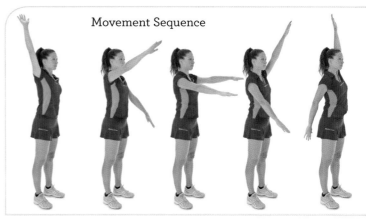

CAUTION
Do the movements with a bit of momentum, but without losing control over the speed and the end of the movement. There will be a slight bounce and stretch at the end of each movement, but excessive momentum and speed reduce control over the exercise and increase the risk of injury. Skip this exercise if you feel any discomfort in your shoulder, especially if this happens when you raise it above 90°.

INDICATION
For relieving discomfort in the muscles that operate the shoulder. This exercise aids with shot techniques by optimizing the range of movement in the shoulder, so it is a good choice for all participants in racket and paddle sports.

Scissors

START
Stand with your feet in line with your shoulders. Raise your arms to 90°, and then cross them in front of your body. Finally, bend your elbows so that your fingers point to the rear.

TECHNIQUE
Move your shoulders in horizontal abduction and straighten your elbows so that the initial position is reversed and your arms uncross and move apart. Continue the frontal abduction as far as you can, and after a little bounce, return to the starting position. Repeat the cycle several times without stopping.

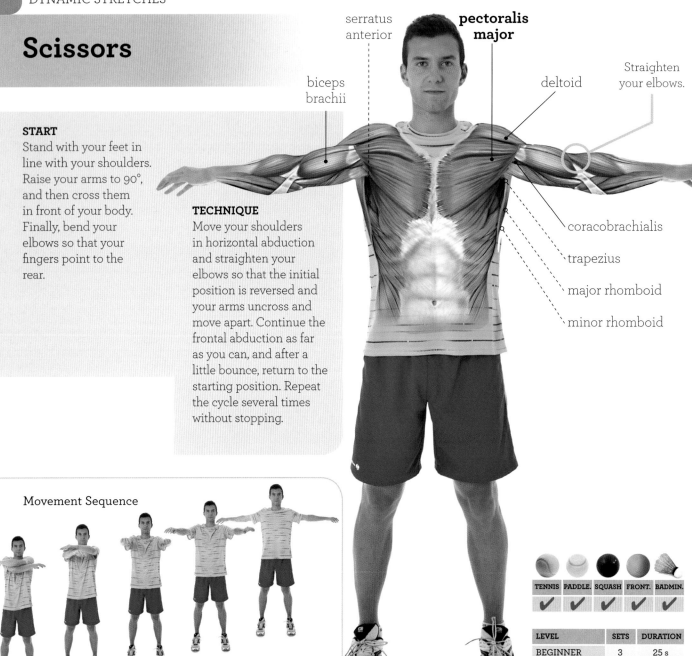

serratus anterior

pectoralis major

biceps brachii

deltoid

Straighten your elbows.

coracobrachialis

trapezius

major rhomboid

minor rhomboid

Movement Sequence

TENNIS	PADDLE.	SQUASH	FRONT.	BADMIN.
✔	✔	✔	✔	✔

LEVEL	SETS	DURATION
BEGINNER	3	25 s
INTERMEDIATE	3	25 s
ADVANCED	4	30 s

CAUTION
Control the speed and force of the bounces to reduce the risk of injury, especially when you reach the end of the movement toward the rear. If you follow this advice and keep a stable position, you will succeed in doing the stretch without any mishaps.

INDICATION
For players of racket and paddle sports because of the relief of muscle tension in the main muscles that operate the shoulder, and because of the optimization of the range of movement in this joint. This will achieve better use of shot strength and technique in both the forehand and the backhand.

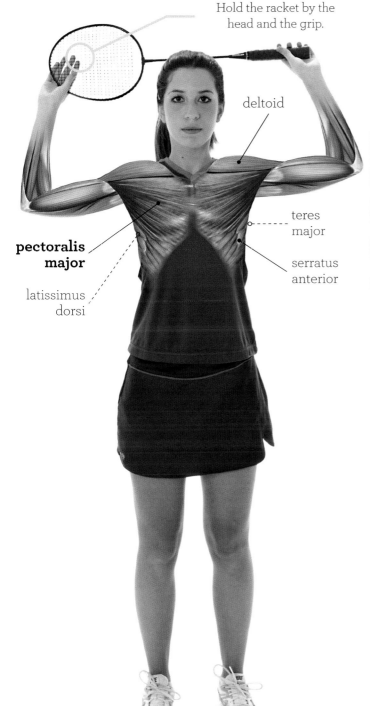

Hold the racket by the head and the grip.

deltoid

teres major

serratus anterior

pectoralis major

latissimus dorsi

Circles with a Racket

START
Grasp a racket with one hand on the head and the other one on the grip. Hold the racket in front of your body using shoulder flexion and keep your elbows straight. Keep your feet slightly separated and your upper body erect.

TECHNIQUE
Move the racket toward one side without changing your grip, so that one shoulder remains in abduction and the opposite forearm is over your head. Continue the circular movement behind your head and then toward your opposite side, and finally return to the starting point. Repeat the cycle several times.

TENNIS	PADDLE.	SQUASH	FRONT.	BADMIN.
✔	✔	✔	✔	✔

LEVEL	SETS	DURATION
BEGINNER	2	20 s
INTERMEDIATE	2	25 s
ADVANCED	3	25 s

Movement Sequence

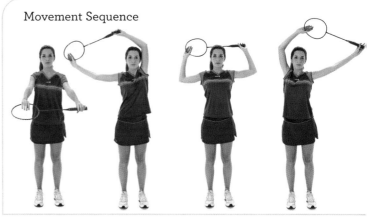

CAUTION
Some parts of this movement require reaching a shoulder position close to the limit of its range of motion. Do the exercise at a moderate speed and keep control at all times so you can stop before experiencing the slightest discomfort, without compromising the integrity of your joints.

INDICATION
For preparing the shoulder joint for play, reaching the optimal range of motion, and fostering good technique, resulting in more fluid play and improving power and accuracy in the various shots.

Side Bend

deltoid

teres major

latissimus dorsi

trapezius

internal oblique

START

Start with your feet at least shoulder width apart. Raise one arm with the palm facing forward, as if you were giving the signal to halt. The other arm remains relaxed.

TECHNIQUE

Bend your upper body toward the side opposite the raised arm. This arm should move over your head while the opposite one moves behind your back. Toward the end of the movement, the raised forearm should be nearly parallel to the floor; try to go as far as possible with your hand. Repeat the movement toward the other side.

Movement Sequence

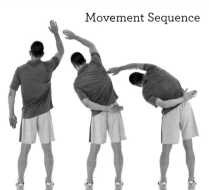
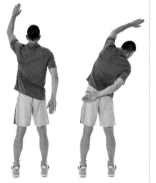

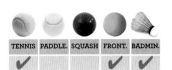

					LEVEL	SETS	DURATION
TENNIS	PADDLE.	SQUASH	FRONT.	BADMIN.	BEGINNER	3	25 s
✔		✔		✔	INTERMEDIATE	3	30 s
					ADVANCED	3	30 s

Keep an adequate spread between your feet.

CAUTION

Keep your feet far enough apart for stable balance. Avoid brusque movements, and prolong the stretch to get the best results with the least possible risk.

INDICATION

For maintaining optimum range of motion in the shoulders, and preparing some of the muscles that operate them for playing. This exercise reduces the risk of injury in subsequent activity, and it helps with the breadth of movement and fluidity in the shots.

Upper-Body Rotation

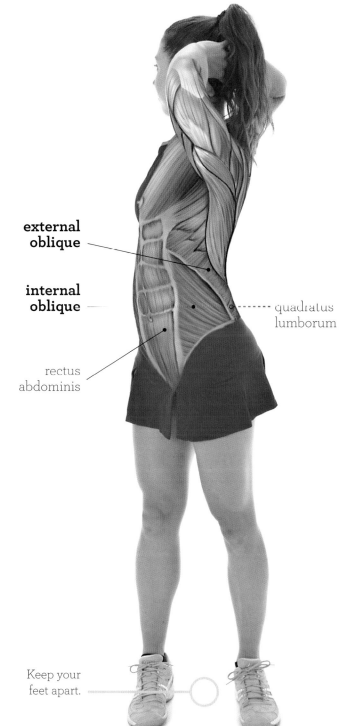

external
oblique

internal
oblique

quadratus
lumborum

rectus
abdominis

Keep your
feet apart.

START

Stand with your feet
shoulder width apart.
Raise your hands and
place them behind your
neck, with your elbows
bent and your shoulders
in abduction. Keep your
shoulders in line with
your hips, and your
upper body erect.

TECHNIQUE

Rotate your upper body
to one side; use a bit of
momentum and a very
gentle bounce that marks
the change in direction as
you rotate toward the other
side. Repeat the movement
toward alternating sides
several times. You will feel
the stretch in the sides of
your upper body.

Movement Sequence

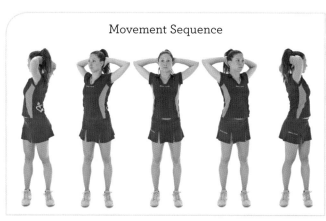

	TENNIS	PADDLE.	SQUASH	FRONT.	BADMIN.
	✔			✔	✔

LEVEL	SETS	DURATION
BEGINNER	2	25 s
INTERMEDIATE	3	25 s
ADVANCED	3	30 s

CAUTION

Remember that if you use any
bounce it should be very gentle,
and even though you should use
slight momentum, the speed will
have to be moderate to keep the
stretch under control at all times
and minimize risks.

INDICATION

Especially for prevention of injuries
to the abdominal muscles in players
in disciplines in which there is a lot
of high play, as in badminton, or
when high shots are powerful, as in
the tennis serve and certain shots in
frontenis.

Slalom

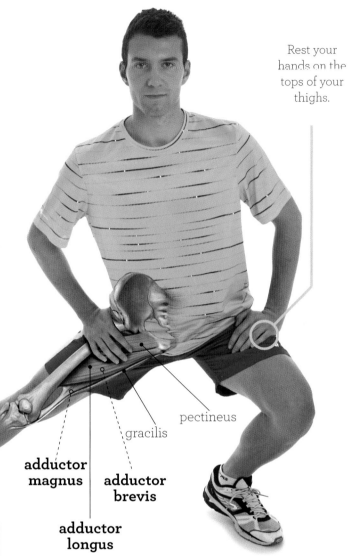

Rest your hands on the tops of your thighs.

START
Stand with your feet far apart. Your knees should be straight, with your upper body erect, and your hands can rest on your upper thighs to help you hold an upper-body position, leaning slightly forward as you do this exercise.

TECHNIQUE
Bend the knee on one side so that your whole body moves in that direction and produces abduction in the opposite hip. Your feet should stay in their original positions without moving. When you reach the end of the movement, change directions and do the movement toward the other side. You will feel the stretch in your groin and the inner face of your thighs.

pectineus

gracilis

adductor magnus

adductor brevis

adductor longus

Movement Sequence

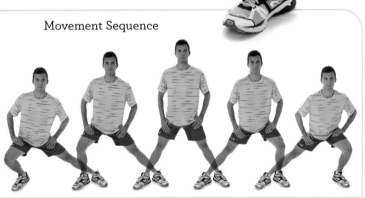

TENNIS	PADDLE.	SQUASH	FRONT.	BADMIN.
✓	✓	✓	✓	✓

LEVEL	SETS	DURATION
BEGINNER	2	20 s
INTERMEDIATE	2	25 s
ADVANCED	2	30 s

CAUTION
Perform the movement at a moderately slow speed so you can brake at the end of the movement with a slight, controlled bounce. Remember that the adductors can easily feel some negative effects if they are stretched too far or they are subjected to strain during play.

INDICATION
In combination with a warm-up, to reduce the risk of injury and improve performance during play. This is highly recommended for running to the side in racket and paddle sports.

Pendulum

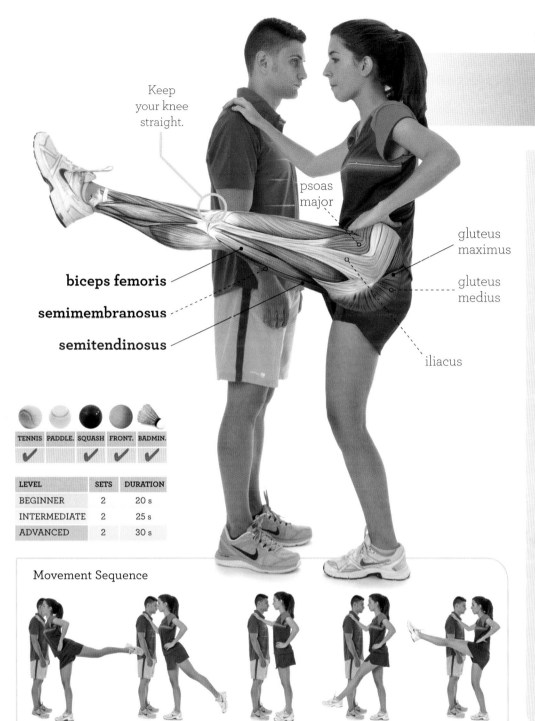

Keep your knee straight.

psoas major

biceps femoris

semimembranosus

semitendinosus

gluteus maximus

gluteus medius

iliacus

TENNIS	PADDLE.	SQUASH	FRONT.	BADMIN.
✔		✔	✔	✔

LEVEL	SETS	DURATION
BEGINNER	2	20 s
INTERMEDIATE	2	25 s
ADVANCED	2	30 s

Movement Sequence

START

Stand beside a partner so that the two of you face opposite directions. Place one hand on the other person's shoulder and your free hand on your waist. Your upper body should be in line with your legs and perpendicular to the floor.

TECHNIQUE

Move your outside leg rearward, raising your foot as high as you can and keeping your knee almost totally straight. When you reach the highest point, change the direction of the movement and swing your leg forward, using the force of gravity until you reach the highest point in front. Then repeat the sequence several times, moving your leg like a pendulum.

CAUTION

It's a good idea to take advantage of momentum to reach the optimum range of motion. The pendulum movement works well as long as you do not use excessive speed, and your bounces are not too abrupt or uncontrolled; otherwise they could be detrimental, especially for the ischiotibial muscles.

INDICATION

For training for running and the jumps performed during a game, plus to relieve tension in the hip flexor and extensor muscles and the knee flexors.

Lateral Pendulum

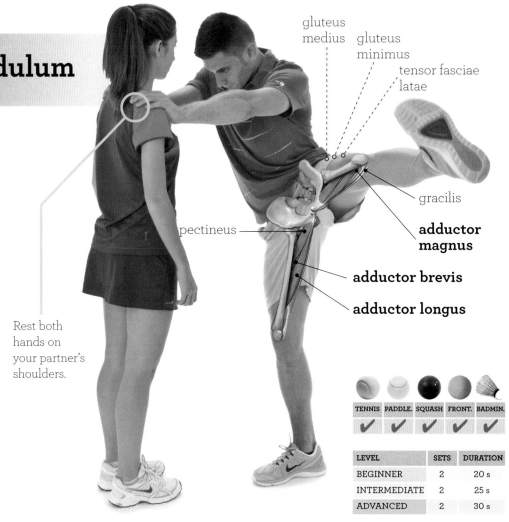

gluteus medius
gluteus minimus
tensor fasciae latae
gracilis
adductor magnus
adductor brevis
adductor longus
pectineus

START
Stand in front of a partner you can use for support. Place your hands on your partner's shoulders and keep your elbows straight to maintain maximum distance from the person. Keep one foot on the floor with the corresponding knee straight as you slightly flex the opposite hip so that your foot rises slightly to the front.

TECHNIQUE
Perform adduction with the bent hip so that your leg crosses in front of the other one as far as possible. When you reach the end, move in the opposite direction until your hip reaches maximum abduction; then repeat the cycle without pausing at the starting position, and prolonging the pendulum movement.

Rest both hands on your partner's shoulders.

TENNIS	PADDLE.	SQUASH	FRONT.	BADMIN.
✔	✔	✔	✔	✔

LEVEL	SETS	DURATION
BEGINNER	2	20 s
INTERMEDIATE	2	25 s
ADVANCED	2	30 s

Movement Sequence

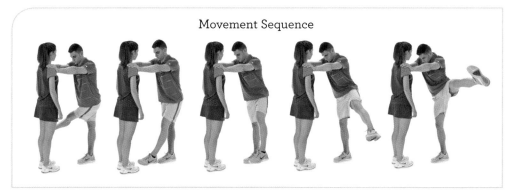

CAUTION
Avoid great acceleration at the end of the stretch, since that would require an abrupt stop and the negative consequences that could result for tendons, muscles, and joints. Always keep the movement under control and go no farther than a very slight bounce when you reach the end of the movement.

INDICATION
For participants in racket or paddle sports, since this exercise involves hip abductor and adductor muscles which are often used in the common pattern of running to the side.

High Skipping

Bend your hip to the maximum.

gluteus maximus

gluteus minimus

START
Stand in a relatively open area; even though this exercise can be done either in place or on the move, you will be moving your arms and legs. Keep your hands and arms relaxed, with your upper body in line with your legs and perpendicular to the floor.

TECHNIQUE
Bend the hip and knee of one leg as you bend the shoulder and elbow on the opposite side. The ankle of your support foot will go into plantar flexion, as if you were striding uphill or jumping. Do the same movement alternatively with both legs and make sure to use enough impetus to achieve the proper range of movement.

TENNIS	PADDLE.	SQUASH	FRONT.	BADMIN.
✔			✔	✔

LEVEL	SETS	DURATION
BEGINNER	3	20 s
INTERMEDIATE	3	25 s
ADVANCED	3	30 s

Movement Sequence

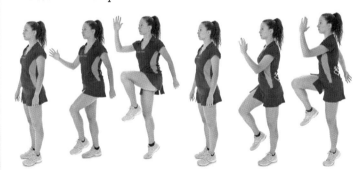

CAUTION
This exercise entails no major risk; even though it is dynamic, the impetus used is not sufficient to endanger the hip or its powerful extensor muscles. Just be careful about moving in an open space and doing the changes in support points carefully.

INDICATION
For players of paddle and racket sports, especially for the ones where starts and sprints are nearly continuous, and for runners of fairly long distances because of the dimensions of the playing field. This also contributes to the warm-up and preparation for athletic participation.

Skip to the Rear

START

Stand with your upper body in line with your legs and perpendicular to the floor. Choose an open area; even though this exercise can be done either in place or on the move, as with the High Skipping, this stretch likewise requires moving the arms and legs.

TECHNIQUE

Extend one hip and bend the corresponding knee as you also slightly bend the shoulder and elbow of the opposite side, as if you were making a running stride. Alternate these movements using both sides as if you were running, but lifting your heels until they make contact behind you; this will stretch primarily the quadriceps femoris.

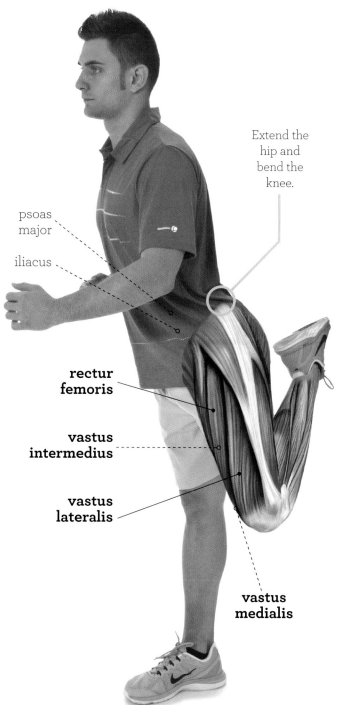

Extend the hip and bend the knee.

psoas major

iliacus

rectur femoris

vastus intermedius

vastus lateralis

vastus medialis

Movement Sequence

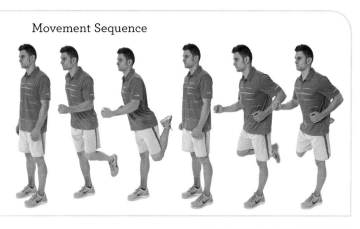

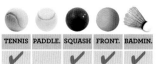

	TENNIS	PADDLE.	SQUASH	FRONT.	BADMIN.
	✓		✓	✓	✓

LEVEL	SETS	DURATION
BEGINNER	3	20 s
INTERMEDIATE	3	25 s
ADVANCED	3	30 s

CAUTION

This dynamic stretch entails no risk and can be done with impetus, in contrast to most of the exercises of this type. Make sure to use an open space so you don't bump into anything, or that you have room in front of you in case you do the exercise on the move.

INDICATION

For participants in racket and paddle sports, especially when running, jumping, and long strides are more important, since these movements place significant demands on the quadriceps femoris and other muscles.

Steps in Pushup Position

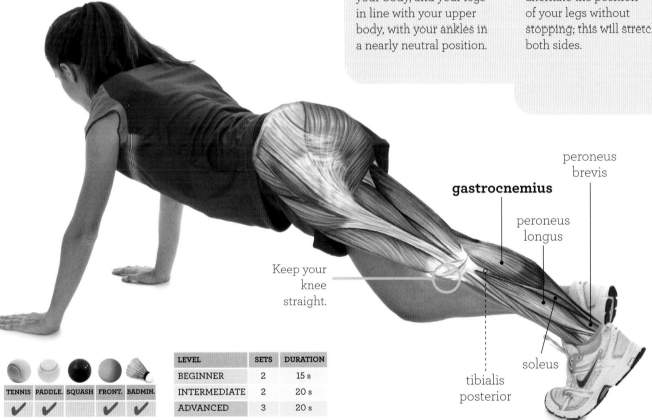

Movement Sequence

START

Get into the plank position, holding yourself up on your hands and your toes, as if you were going to do a pushup. Your elbows should be straight, your shoulders about perpendicular to your body, and your legs in line with your upper body, with your ankles in a nearly neutral position.

TECHNIQUE

Slightly bend one knee and shift your weight to the opposite leg; the corresponding ankle will move into dorsal flexion, which will produce the stretch in the plantar flexors. Continually alternate the position of your legs without stopping; this will stretch both sides.

peroneus brevis

gastrocnemius

peroneus longus

Keep your knee straight.

soleus

tibialis posterior

		LEVEL	SETS	DURATION
		BEGINNER	2	15 s
		INTERMEDIATE	2	20 s
		ADVANCED	3	20 s

TENNIS	PADDLE.	SQUASH	FRONT.	BADMIN.
✔	✔		✔	✔

CAUTION

Maintain the natural curvature of your spine and don't let your body sag toward the floor because of the weight being supported. This will protect your back and make you work your abdominal muscles isometrically.

INDICATION

To relieve the strain that many athletes in racket and paddle sports may experience in the calf muscles as a result of repeated fast starts and sprints, and to prevent problems common to these sports, such as rupture of the medial head of the gastrocnemius or tennis leg.

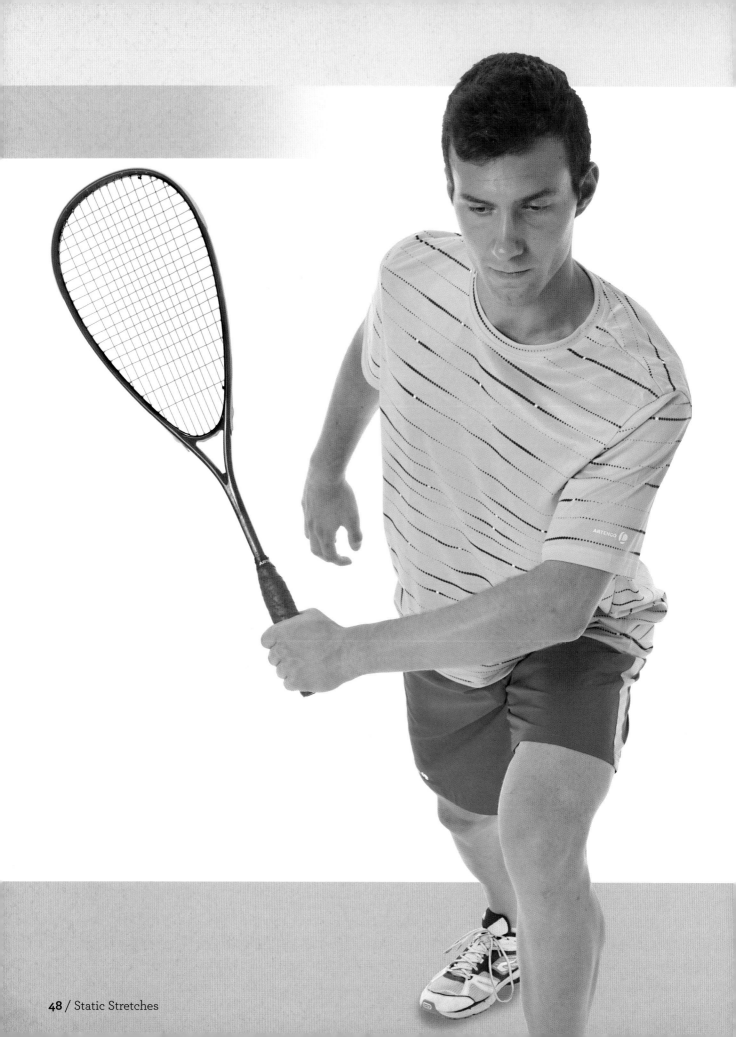

STATIC
STRETCHES

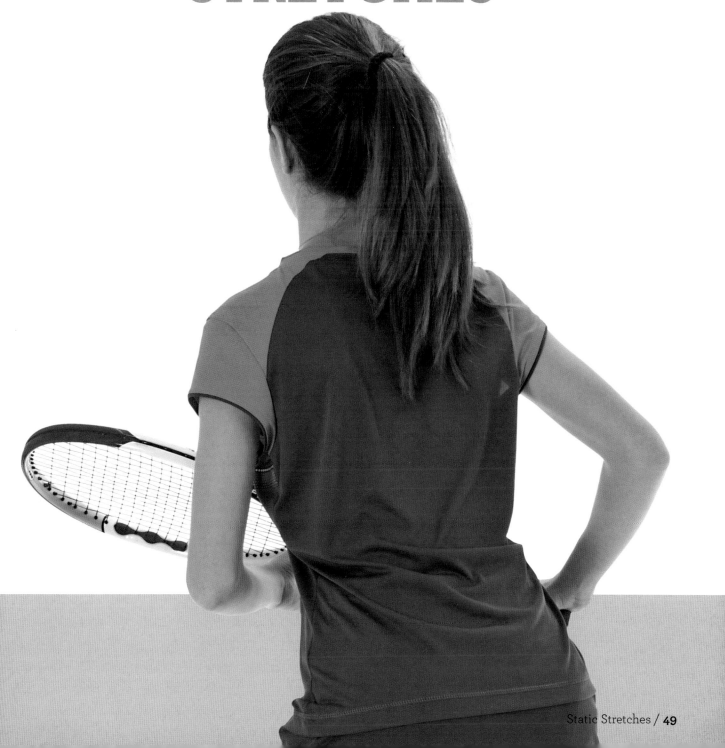

THE BASICS OF STATIC STRETCHES

Static stretches surely are the most popular ones that traditionally have been associated with athletic activity. Even though they are not the best choice for a warm-up prior to training or competition, as we saw in the previous section, except for a few disciplines such as rhythmic gymnastics, they can indeed be very helpful when done at other times.

Static stretches have proven to be more effective when the purpose is to achieve the broadest possible range of movement, especially the passive stretches and ones done using proprioceptive neuromuscular facilitation (PNF). There may also be some advantages at certain times related to competition. For example, if an athlete feels muscle strain or extreme fatigue during a break in competition, some gentle stretching combined with massage on the area may make it possible to face the next period or match successfully, as we often see in breaks during tennis matches.

Static stretches done following athletic activity, particularly in sports where significant muscle congestion occurs in training or competition, as in 4 × 400 m races, and strength and hypertrophy sports, may encourage replenishment of blood to the muscles, and thus bring more oxygen and nutrients to the muscles. This surely will encourage at least partial recovery in the muscles involved.

On the other hand, stretching sessions not related to athletics, in other words, ones done in isolation, are a good way to increase flexibility and encourage relaxation. In such instances we should remember that every stretching session should be preceded by a warm-up, no matter how brief, for the intended muscles, since they need to be brought up to speed before subjecting them to the tension involved in static stretches. In any case, if we play a racket or paddle sport, extreme flexibility can turn out to be counterproductive, as in any other sport where the movements are performed quickly, with lots of force, or both together. The result of that may be joint instability, which would not be appropriate in a

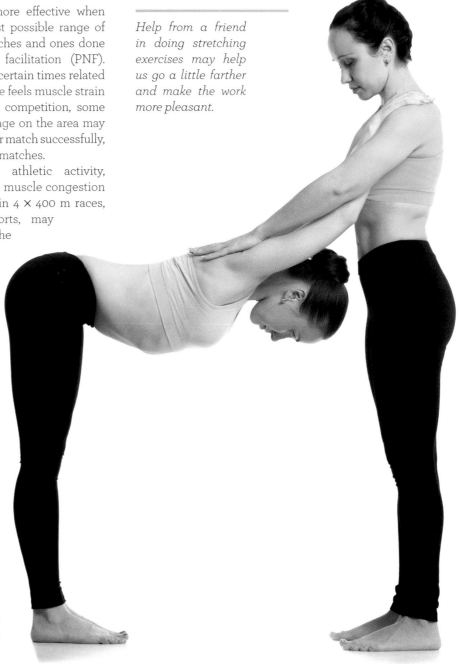

Help from a friend in doing stretching exercises may help us go a little farther and make the work more pleasant.

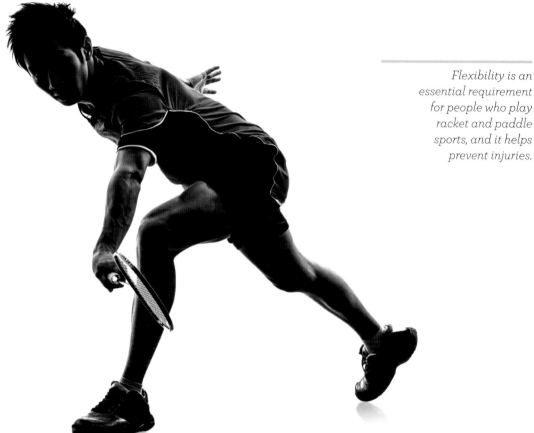

Flexibility is an essential requirement for people who play racket and paddle sports, and it helps prevent injuries.

sport where joint stability is crucial for repeatedly hitting the ball and performing the backswing followed by the forehand swing.

Sometimes sports are played in groups or in the company of a friend, as a couple, or with a trainer. This may make it possible to do assisted stretches: a friend helps in performing the stretch, in order to go a little farther than what is possible when exercising alone.

In theory this is positive, but you have to be sure that your helper knows how to assist, and that you remain in constant communication. Clear communication and the appropriate execution speed will greatly reduce the risk of injury. It goes without saying that pulling and joking have to be put aside until after the game, and never done while assisting a friend in a stretch, since the results could be catastrophic.

There are several points that must be kept in mind while doing the stretches:

■ Static stretches lasting from 15 to 30 seconds have proven to be the most effective ones for increasing flexibility, although some experts recommend durations of up to 60 seconds, especially for very powerful muscle groups.

■ A stretch can be done several times in a single session, as long as there is enough rest time between sets.

■ Improving flexibility, like any other progress in physical activity, comes gradually, so overdoing the intensity of the stretches will not produce faster progress, but almost certainly an injury.

■ Setting priorities is essential, since not all muscles in the body exhibit the same degree of stiffness or flexibility. Focusing on the muscles that already are more flexible, or overlooking the stiffest ones, will lead to reduced fluidity and precision in running and making shots.

Finally, we need to remember that stretching should be done with warmed-up muscles, regardless of the chosen timing for the stretching session, and that the combination of warm-up and stretching will always produce better results than stretches done in isolation, whether dynamic or static.

UPPER-BODY AND NECK STRETCHES

In racket and paddle sports, the neck and upper-body muscles are called on for many reasons. The ready position involves leaning the upper body forward and isometric work in the spinal erectors to keep the back straight. Moves such as a tennis serve and an overhead involve extension of the spine during the backswing, followed by a rapid contraction at the time of the shot. This requires the muscles used in the extension and the flexion of the upper body to straighten and contract abruptly and in a very short time, so it is essential that they be well trained. The muscles used in the adduction of the scapula work during the backswing for forehand and backhand shots. The latter also involves considerable rotation in the upper body, especially when both hands are used, so they too need to be prepared to withstand great tension and intensity.

RHOMBOIDS

The rhomboideus major and minor are next to one another and act as a functional unit, and they are stretched in the same way. The function of both muscles is the retraction and the raising of the scapula.

Rhomboideus Major: This muscle originates at the spiny apophyses of vertebrae T1 to T4, and it inserts at the medial edge of the scapula.

Rhomboideus Minor: This muscle originates at the spiny apophyses of vertebrae C6 and C7, and it inserts at the medial edge of the scapula above the insertion of the rhomboideus major.

TRAPEZIUS

This muscle has a broad origin, from the superior nuchal line of the occipital bone, passing through the nuchal ligament and the spiny apophyses of vertebrae C7 to T12. Its insertion is located at the lateral third of the clavicle, the acromion, and the scapular spine. In this section we are particularly interested in the descending part of this muscle, for among its functions is the extension of the head and the spinal column.

SEMISPINALIS

The entire muscle spans from the occipital bone to the transverse apophysis of vertebra T12.

Its bilateral contraction produces extension of the head and the cervical and thoracic vertebrae, and its unilateral contraction tilts and rotates the head and the cervical and thoracic vertebrae.

ILIOCOSTALIS

The iliocostalis muscle spans from the sacral bone to the transverse apophyses of vertebrae C4 to C6 and can be divided into three parts:

Cervical Iliocostalis: This muscle originates at ribs 3 through 7, and it inserts at the transverse apophyses of vertebrae C4 to C6.

Thoracic Iliocostalis: This muscle originates at ribs 7 to 12, and inserts at ribs 1 through 6.

Lumbar Iliocostalis: This muscle originates at the sacral bone, the iliac crest, and the thoracolumbar fascia, and inserts at ribs 7 to 12.

It is part of the paravertebral muscles, so its main function is extension of the spine, although when it is used unilaterally it tilts it to one side.

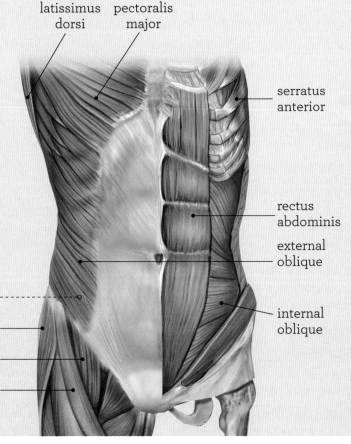

latissimus dorsi
pectoralis major
serratus anterior
rectus abdominis
external oblique
internal oblique
quadratus lumborum
tensor fasciae latae
iliopsoas
sartorius

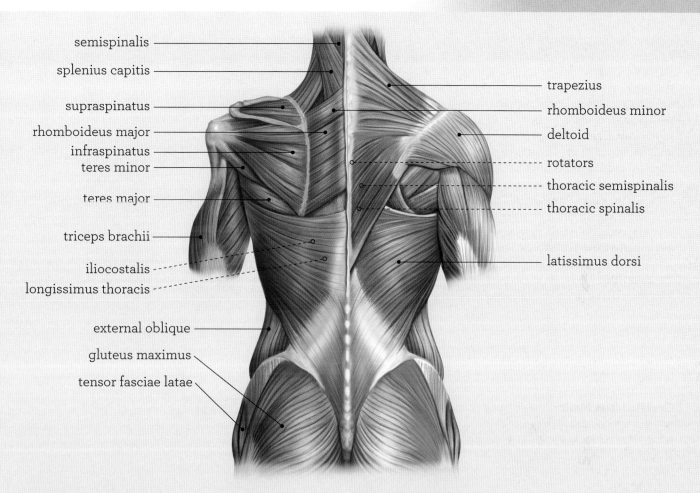

semispinalis

splenius capitis

supraspinatus

rhomboideus major

infraspinatus

teres minor

teres major

triceps brachii

iliocostalis

longissimus thoracis

external oblique

gluteus maximus

tensor fasciae latae

trapezius

rhomboideus minor

deltoid

rotators

thoracic semispinalis

thoracic spinalis

latissimus dorsi

LONGISSIMUS THORACIS

The longissimus thoracis spans from the sacral bone to the mastoid apophysis of the temporal bone, and it is divided into three parts:

Longissimus Capitis: This muscle originates at the transverse apophyses of vertebrae T1 to T3 and the transverse and articular apophyses of vertebrae C4 to C7. It inserts at the mastoid apophysis of the temporal bone.

Longissimus Cervicis: This muscle originates at the transverse apophyses of vertebrae T1 to T6 and inserts at the transverse apophyses of vertebrae C2 to C5.

Longissimus Thoracis: This muscle originates at the sacral bone, the iliac crest, and the spiny apophysis of vertebrae L1 to L5. It inserts at ribs 2 to 12, the transverse apophyses of vertebrae T1 to T12 and the costal apophyses of vertebrae L1 to L5.

Bilateral contraction of the longissimus capitis extends the head; its unilateral contraction turns it. The longissimus cervicis and thoracis extend the spine when they work bilaterally, and bend it to the side when they work unilaterally.

RECTUS ABDOMINIS

This muscle originates at the pubic crest and symphysis, and inserts at the xiphoid process and the cartilage of ribs 5 to 7. Its functions are flexion of the upper body and compression of the abdomen.

EXTERNAL OBLIQUE

This muscle originates at ribs 5 to 12 and inserts at the linea alba, the os pubis, and the iliac crest. Its functions are bending and rotating the upper body when used unilaterally, and flexing the upper body and compressing the abdomen when it is used bilaterally.

INTERNAL OBLIQUE

This muscle originates at the thoracolumbar fascia, the iliac crest, and the inguinal ligament, and it inserts at ribs 10 to 12 and the linea alba. Bilateral contraction bends the upper body and compresses the abdomen, and unilateral contraction bends and rotates the upper body.

Rear Arm Pull

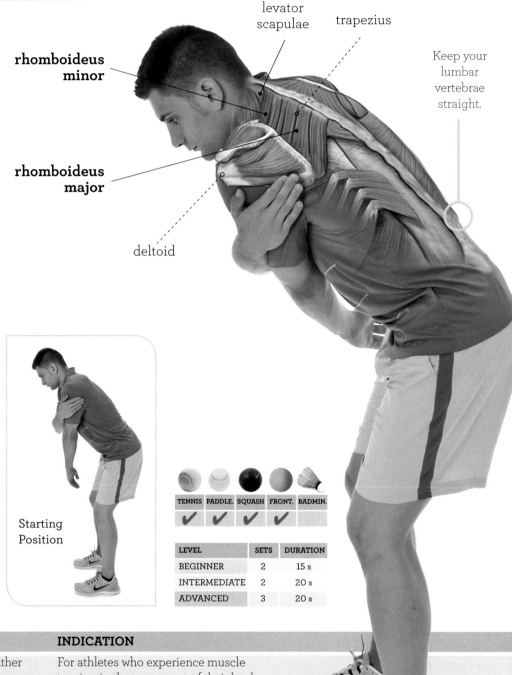

levator scapulae

trapezius

rhomboideus minor

rhomboideus major

deltoid

Keep your lumbar vertebrae straight.

START

Stand with your knees slightly bent and your upper body leaning forward. Protect your back by maintaining the natural curvature of your spine. Let one arm hang down, and place your other hand between your upper arm and the back of your shoulder so that you have a firm grip.

TECHNIQUE

While keeping the same position with your hand, pull on your arm and try to achieve frontal adduction. The arm being pulled should end up crossing in front of your chest and produce scapular abduction, which is necessary for stretching the rhomboideus muscles. You will feel muscle tension in your back on the side of the arm being pulled, and near your thoracic vertebrae.

Starting Position

TENNIS	PADDLE.	SQUASH	FRONT.	BADMIN.
✔	✔	✔	✔	

LEVEL	SETS	DURATION
BEGINNER	2	15 s
INTERMEDIATE	2	20 s
ADVANCED	3	20 s

CAUTION

Focus on scapular abduction rather than solely on frontal adduction of the arm; this is the only way to assure an efficient stretch. You will have to pull hard if you want to feel the tension, since the muscles involved are powerful ones, and they put up significant resistance.

INDICATION

For athletes who experience muscle tension in the upper part of their back due to the high demands placed on the scapular adductor muscles in both the backswing for forehand shots and the advance and impact from backhand shots. This stretch is also a good choice for general training and injury prevention in racket sports.

Starting Position

Seated Leg Pull

START
Sit down with your back erect and bend your hips and knees to bring your thighs close to your chest. Your knees should remain together, with the soles of your feet resting on the floor. Place your forearms under your knees and firmly grasp your elbows.

TECHNIQUE
Try to pull with your upper body, without moving your legs, and keep holding on to your elbows. The middle of your back should arch to the rear while your shoulders remain forward and your chest hollowed. This movement produces scapular abduction and stretches the rhomboideus muscles.

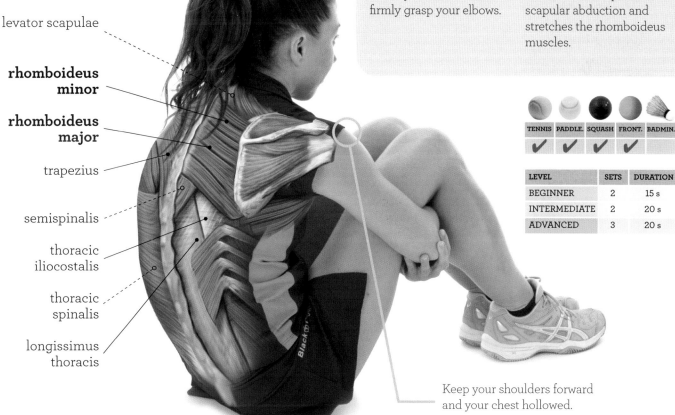

	TENNIS	PADDLE.	SQUASH	FRONT.	BADMIN.
	✔	✔	✔	✔	

LEVEL	SETS	DURATION
BEGINNER	2	15 s
INTERMEDIATE	2	20 s
ADVANCED	3	20 s

levator scapulae

rhomboideus minor

rhomboideus major

trapezius

semispinalis

thoracic iliocostalis

thoracic spinalis

longissimus thoracis

Keep your shoulders forward and your chest hollowed.

CAUTION
Concentrate on arching the upper and middle part of your back outward, and remember that the important part is the scapular abduction: bending the upper body, which permits stretching the spinal erectors, is secondary in this instance.

INDICATION
For athletes who feel sustained muscle tension in the top of their back, or who want to prevent it. This tension results from the high demands placed on the rhomboideus muscles in the backswing for a forehand shot and in the acceleration phase prior to a backhand. It is also indicated as part of general athletic training.

Self-assisted Side Neck Bend

START

Stand with your back erect and your feet shoulder width apart. Place one hand on top of your head with your fingers pointing to the ear on the opposite side so you can apply light posterior traction. Place your free hand behind your back at the height of your lumbar vertebrae and with your palm facing rearward.

TECHNIQUE

Pull your head and neck to the side. At the same time, slide your other hand on your lumbar region along a descending diagonal line. The combination of these two movements will maximize the stretch in the trapezius muscle, and you will feel the tension from the stretch right away.

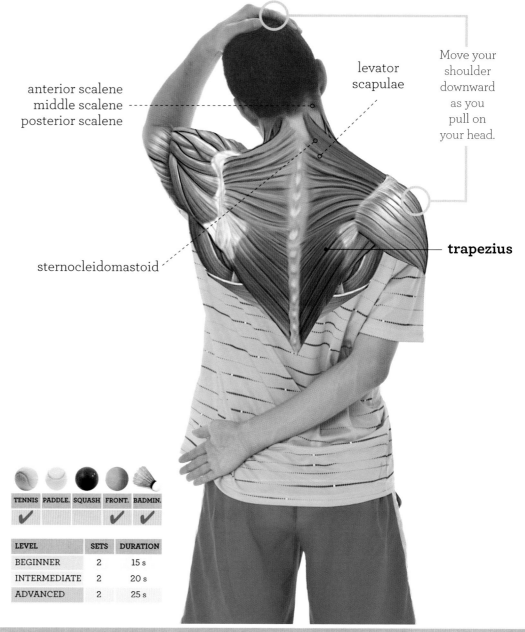

anterior scalene
middle scalene
posterior scalene

levator scapulae

Move your shoulder downward as you pull on your head.

trapezius

sternocleidomastoid

TENNIS	PADDLE.	SQUASH	FRONT.	BADMIN.
✔			✔	✔

LEVEL	SETS	DURATION
BEGINNER	2	15 s
INTERMEDIATE	2	20 s
ADVANCED	2	25 s

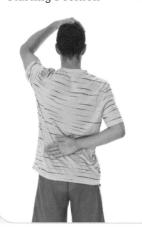

Starting Position

CAUTION

Be careful in pulling on your head and remember that your spinal column is very sensitive to pulling and pushing forces. If you feel any discomfort in this area, stop doing the stretch or reduce the intensity.

INDICATION

For any player of racket or paddle sports because of the use of the trapezius in the backswing for the forehand shot, the advance in the backhand, and holding the paddle or racket in the ready position for a long time. It is especially recommended for players of tennis, frontenis, and badminton because of the many high shots that require using the trapezius muscle in the backswing.

Side Neck Bend with Racket

anterior scalene
middle scalene
posterior scalene

sternocleidomastoid

levator scapulae

trapezius

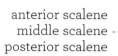

Starting Position

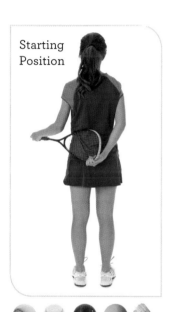

TENNIS	PADDLE.	SQUASH	FRONT.	BADMIN.
✔		✔	✔	

LEVEL	SETS	DURATION
BEGINNER	2	15 s
INTERMEDIATE	2	20 s
ADVANCED	3	20 s

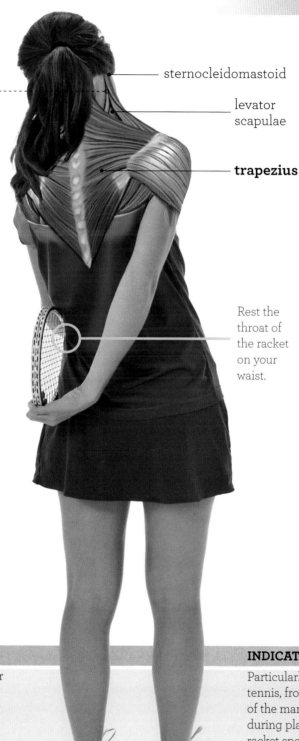

Rest the throat of the racket on your waist.

START
Stand and hold the racket with one hand on the grip. Reverse your customary hold so that the head of the racket points to the rear, and the throat is about waist height. Put your free hand behind your back and hold the frame of the racket firmly.

TECHNIQUE
Bend your head and neck to the side where the racket is. Push the grip toward the inside so that it pivots on your waist, and the hand holding the frame moves farther away from the centerline of your body. The tilt in your head and neck, along with the simultaneous lowering of your shoulder, will stretch the trapezius muscle; you will feel the stretch easily.

CAUTION
This exercise involves no particular risk, but be sure to hold the racket firmly with both hands, that it pivots correctly, and that holding the position causes no discomfort in the hip support or the hand holding the frame.

INDICATION
Particularly recommended for players of tennis, frontenis, and badminton because of the many high shots that are required during play; also for any participant in racket sports because of the involvement of the trapezius in the backswing for the forehand shot, the advance and shot in the backhand, and holding the ready position.

Self-assisted Neck Bend

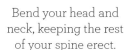

Bend your head and neck, keeping the rest of your spine erect.

START
Stand with your feet a comfortable distance apart and your upper body perpendicular to the floor. Your neck should remain erect, with your gaze straight ahead. Raise your hands and place them so that they hold your head from behind. You can lock your fingers together if that is more comfortable.

TECHNIQUE
Gently pull your head to the front to produce flexion in your head and neck. Even though the tension from the stretch may not be very noticeable, this movement and holding the final position will stretch the extensor muscles of the head and neck.

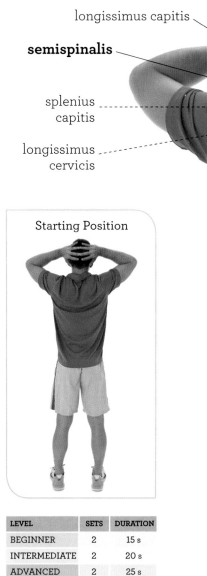

Starting Position

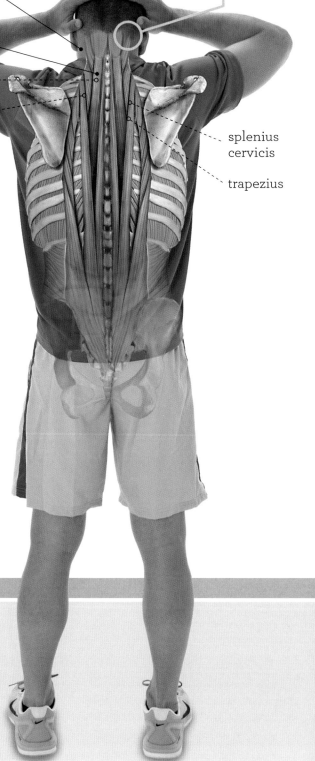

longissimus capitis

semispinalis

splenius capitis

longissimus cervicis

splenius cervicis

trapezius

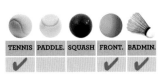

	TENNIS	PADDLE.	SQUASH	FRONT.	BADMIN.
	✔			✔	✔

LEVEL	SETS	DURATION
BEGINNER	2	15 s
INTERMEDIATE	2	20 s
ADVANCED	2	25 s

CAUTION
The cervical vertebrae are sensitive to any kind of force applied to them, so be careful in performing the traction and do not use excessive force. If you feel any discomfort, stop doing the exercise or reduce the intensity.

INDICATION
Particularly for athletes who experience muscle discomfort in the back of the neck, and for players who keep their head and neck in extension for long periods of time in a ready position with their upper body leaning forward, or because of the number of high balls during play.

Neck Bend and Rotation

longissimus capitis

semispinalis

splenius capitis

splenius cervicis

trapezius

longissimus cervicis

levator scapulae

Lower your head and tilt it to one side.

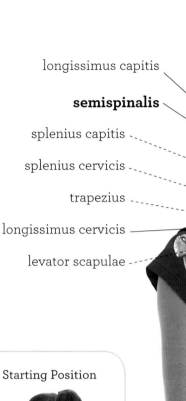

Starting Position

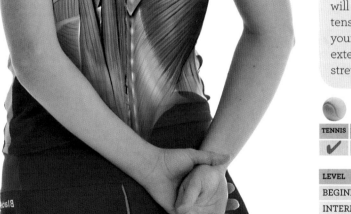

START
Stand with your upper body and neck erect and your gaze straight ahead. Place both hands behind your back or at your sides, with both arms relaxed. Keep your feet a comfortable distance apart.

TECHNIQUE
Lower your head and tilt it, trying to move your chin close to the areas of your pectorals and deltoids. Extend the movement as far as possible, and keep applying pressure when you reach the end. You will feel slight muscle tension in the back of your neck, but to a lesser extent than with other stretches.

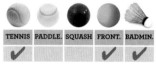

TENNIS	PADDLE.	SQUASH	FRONT.	BADMIN.
✔		✔	✔	

LEVEL	SETS	DURATION
BEGINNER	2	15 s
INTERMEDIATE	3	20 s
ADVANCED	3	25 s

CAUTION
Even though the movement and the stretch seem slight, they will be adequate, and you need not add any other movements to the technique described, such as advancing a shoulder or bending your upper body, since they will contribute no effectiveness to the exercise.

INDICATION
For athletes who feel muscle discomfort in the back of the neck, and for players who use a ready position with the upper body leaning sharply forward, or who play paddle or racket sports involving lots of high balls, because of the movements in the neck extensor muscles.

Upper-Body Bend on Stool

START

Sit on a stool, a low bench, or something similar that is relatively low and lets you rest both feet on the floor without having to straighten your knees beyond 110°. Lean your upper body forward using a slight bend in your hips and keeping your spine straight. Place your arms between your legs with your hands toward the floor and your fingers straight.

TECHNIQUE

Slide the tips of your fingers across the floor and toward the stool by bending your upper body while limiting the bend in your hips. Try to reach as far back as possible so that the upper part of your back is curved. If you perform the exercise properly you will feel the muscle tension on both sides of your thoracic vertebrae.

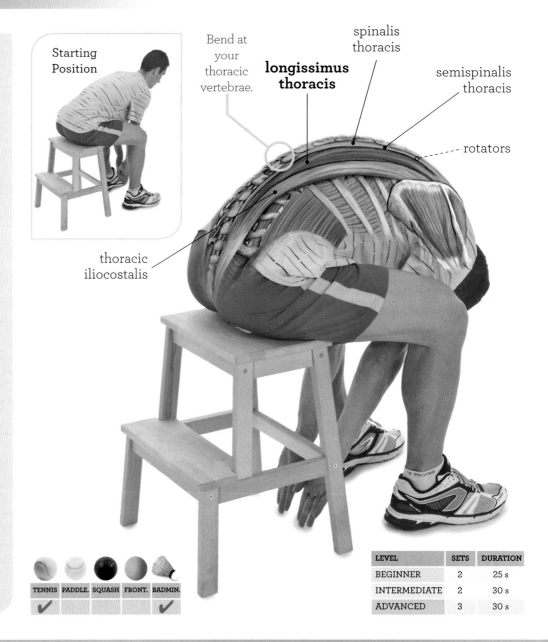

Starting Position

Bend at your thoracic vertebrae.

longissimus thoracis

spinalis thoracis

semispinalis thoracis

rotators

thoracic iliocostalis

	TENNIS	PADDLE.	SQUASH	FRONT.	BADMIN.
	✔				✔

LEVEL	SETS	DURATION
BEGINNER	2	25 s
INTERMEDIATE	2	30 s
ADVANCED	3	30 s

CAUTION

Focus more on bending your thoracic spine and pay less attention to your hips and lumbar spine, since they do not contribute to the main purpose of the stretch. Be sure to use a solid seat and keep your balance as you do the exercise.

INDICATION

Especially for tennis players because of the force from the spinal erectors in the serve, and for badminton players because of the repeated extensions of the spine required by high shots. Also for general training, to relax the tension in the paravertebral muscles, and for players who regularly use a two-handed backhand shot.

Cat Position

Starting Position

spinalis thoracis

Maintain the bend in your thoracic vertebrae

semispinalis thoracis

longissimus thoracis

iliocosta-listhoracis

rhomboideus minor

rhomboideus major

rotators

START

Get down on all fours, with your supporting hands in line with your shoulders and your knees directly beneath your hips. Your knees should be bent at 90° and your elbows should be almost totally straight. Keep your back in a natural position, without letting it sag due to gravity.

TECHNIQUE

Bend your thoracic spine. To do this you will have to pull in your chest and keep your shoulders forward, trying to move the center of your spine upward, as if you were trying to create a hump. When you reach the end of the movement, hold the tension and you will feel the stretch in your paravertebral muscles and the scapular adductors located on each side of the spine.

TENNIS	PADDLE.	SQUASH	FRONT.	BADMIN.
✔				✔

LEVEL	SETS	DURATION
BEGINNER	2	20 s
INTERMEDIATE	2	25 s
ADVANCED	2	30 s

CAUTION

To the extent possible, limit the bend in your thoracic spine, involving as little as possible the lumbar and cervical regions; we will stretch those muscles with other exercises. It's a good idea to use a mat to avoid discomfort in your knees.

INDICATION

For players who feel tension in the thoracic paravertebral muscles, particularly tennis and badminton players, because of the effects of high shots and serving. Also for players of other paddle or racket sports as part of their general training.

Standing Upper-Body Bend

START

Stand with your feet shoulder width apart. Slightly bend your knees and lean your upper body forward, keeping your spine straight. Rest your hands on your knees so that they support you and relieve tension in your lumbar vertebrae.

TECHNIQUE

While maintaining your original supports, bend your upper body, especially in the thoracic region, and try to project the middle of your back outward. To do this you will have to pull in your chest as much as possible while keeping your shoulders forward. Hold the position and you will note a slight stretching sensation in your thoracic paravertebral muscles.

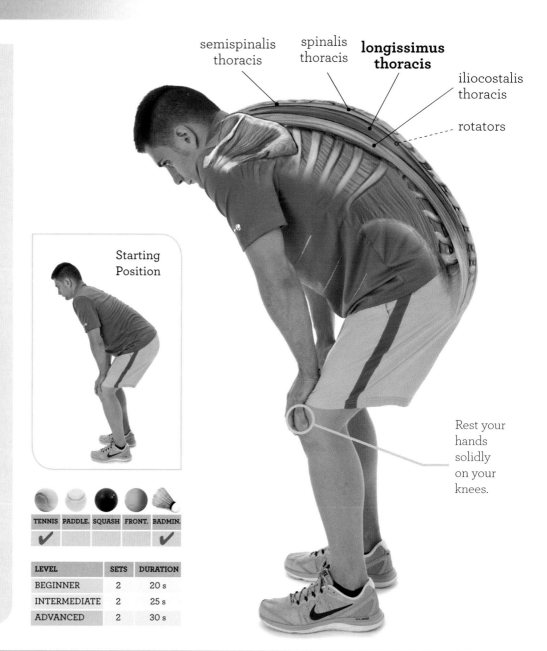

Starting Position

semispinalis thoracis

spinalis thoracis

longissimus thoracis

iliocostalis thoracis

rotators

Rest your hands solidly on your knees.

TENNIS	PADDLE.	SQUASH	FRONT.	BADMIN.
✔				✔

LEVEL	SETS	DURATION
BEGINNER	2	20 s
INTERMEDIATE	2	25 s
ADVANCED	2	30 s

CAUTION

Make sure you have a solid support on your knees which reduces the significant load on the lumbar vertebrae because of the lean in your upper body. This will avoid the discomfort in the lower part of the back that is very common in players of racket sports.

INDICATION

For tennis and badminton players because of the effects of the tennis serve and high play on the paravertebral muscles. Also, though to a lesser degree, for players of paddle or racket sports who want to include this exercise in their training routines as a way to prevent discomfort in the back muscles.

Upper-Body Bend

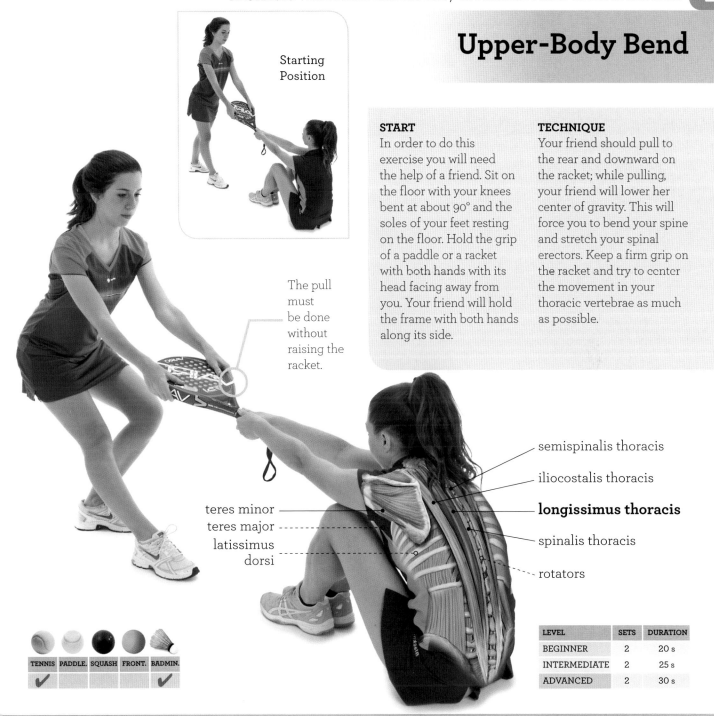

Starting Position

The pull must be done without raising the racket.

START
In order to do this exercise you will need the help of a friend. Sit on the floor with your knees bent at about 90° and the soles of your feet resting on the floor. Hold the grip of a paddle or a racket with both hands with its head facing away from you. Your friend will hold the frame with both hands along its side.

TECHNIQUE
Your friend should pull to the rear and downward on the racket; while pulling, your friend will lower her center of gravity. This will force you to bend your spine and stretch your spinal erectors. Keep a firm grip on the racket and try to center the movement in your thoracic vertebrae as much as possible.

semispinalis thoracis

iliocostalis thoracis

longissimus thoracis

teres minor
teres major
latissimus dorsi

spinalis thoracis

rotators

TENNIS	PADDLE.	SQUASH	FRONT.	BADMIN.
✓				✓

LEVEL	SETS	DURATION
BEGINNER	2	20 s
INTERMEDIATE	2	25 s
ADVANCED	2	30 s

CAUTION
Make sure you communicate continually with your companion and that the pull is gentle and gradual, and never excessive. This, plus proper performance of the technique, will protect your lumbar vertebrae and avoid any possible discomfort.

INDICATION
For players of badminton, tennis, and to a lesser degree, frontenis, because of the serves, high play, and powerful shots, all of which involve the spinal erector muscles. Also for players of other disciplines in which these muscles are used to a greater or lesser degree.

Seated Upper-Body Bend

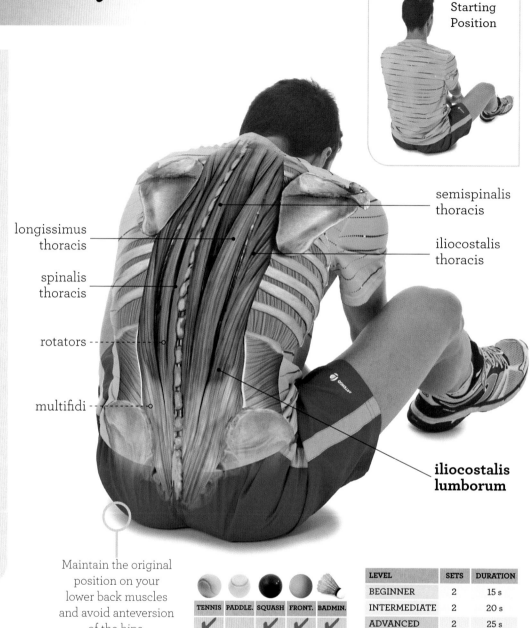

Starting Position

START
Sit down with your upper body perpendicular to the floor, and bend your knees slightly. Hold your legs apart and contact the floor with your heels. Move both arms forward and straighten your elbows so that your forearms are in the open space between your legs, and your fingers point forward and down.

TECHNIQUE
Bend your upper body forward until the pads of your fingers touch the floor; slide them forward. Emphasize the upper body bend to the front and keep your lower back muscles in contact with the floor, avoiding anteversion of the hips. Also keep your heels on the floor and do not change the initial position of your legs.

longissimus thoracis

spinalis thoracis

rotators

multifidi

semispinalis thoracis

iliocostalis thoracis

iliocostalis lumborum

Maintain the original position on your lower back muscles and avoid anteversion of the hips.

TENNIS	PADDLE.	SQUASH	FRONT.	BADMIN.
✔		✔	✔	✔

LEVEL	SETS	DURATION
BEGINNER	2	15 s
INTERMEDIATE	2	20 s
ADVANCED	2	25 s

CAUTION
This exercise stretches the lumbar and thoracic spinal erector muscles, and it may cause some discomfort, especially in the lumbar region, especially if there is some pre-existing problem. If this applies to you, stop the stretch or reduce the intensity.

INDICATION
For players of racket sports in general, but especially for those who feel muscle tension in the lumbar region or who make lots of high, powerful shots, very low shots, and backhand shots, especially with two hands, because of the force exerted by the lumbar muscles and the compression, torsion, and shearing forces that act on the spinal column.

Cringe Position

Starting Position

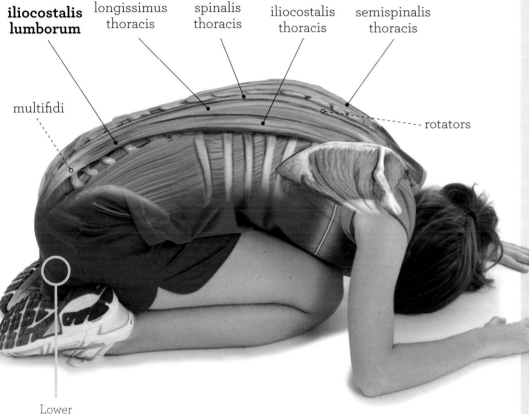

iliocostalis lumborum

longissimus thoracis

spinalis thoracis

iliocostalis thoracis

semispinalis thoracis

multifidi

rotators

Lower your gluteal muscles toward the floor.

TENNIS	PADDLE.	SQUASH	FRONT.	BADMIN.
✔		✔	✔	✔

LEVEL	SETS	DURATION
BEGINNER	2	20 s
INTERMEDIATE	2	25 s
ADVANCED	3	25 s

START
Get down on all fours, with your hands aligned with your shoulders and your knees slightly ahead of your hips. Your ankles should be in plantar flexion so that your insteps are practically touching the floor and your toes are in contact with it.

TECHNIQUE
Bend your knees so that your upper body moves rearward and lowers onto the rear of your thighs and you make contact with your calves. You will also have to bend your elbows and lower your lower back muscles between your heels. Perform retroversion with your hips, accompanied by a bend in your lumbar vertebrae. Some slight contractions of your abdominal muscles while you maintain the position will add to the stretch.

CAUTION
Even though this exercise stretches the spinal erectors, there is no discomfort to the spine because the many support points reduce the pressure on it. You merely need to pay attention to the maximum plantar flexion in your ankles and the weight they support. If you feel any discomfort, separate your feet slightly and reduce the degree of plantar flexion.

INDICATION
For athletes who experience abnormal muscle tension in the lumbar muscles, and for players of disciplines that involve high shots, including the tennis serve, very low shots, or powerful backhands, especially with two hands, because of the attendant extensions and rotations of the spine.

Upper-Body Rotation on All Fours

START

Get down on all fours, with your upper body parallel to the floor; keep your knees slightly apart for added stability in the position. Move one of your hands so that the fingers are slightly forward of your head, but not so far that your arms loses its support function; as you do the exercise it will be the only upper limb that performs this task.

TECHNIQUE

Turn the rearmost hand onto its edge with your fingers pointing toward the opposite side. Slide this hand in the direction signaled by your fingers; this will cause your shoulder to lower and your upper body to rotate. Extend the movement as far as possible, holding yourself up with the forward hand and both knees. You will feel the tension differently in the various areas of your back; it may be more noticeable in the latissimus dorsi than in the lumbar muscles.

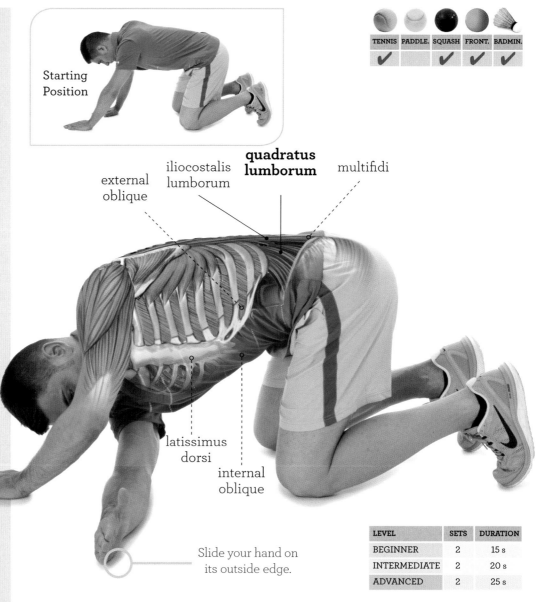

Starting Position

external oblique

iliocostalis lumborum

quadratus lumborum

multifidi

latissimus dorsi

internal oblique

Slide your hand on its outside edge.

	TENNIS	PADDLE.	SQUASH	FRONT.	BADMIN.
	✔		✔	✔	✔

LEVEL	SETS	DURATION
BEGINNER	2	15 s
INTERMEDIATE	2	20 s
ADVANCED	2	25 s

CAUTION

As you do this exercise, make sure that the three permanent support points are solid, and that your knees are far enough apart to keep your balance in the last part of the movement.

INDICATION

For athletes who experience muscle tension in the lumbar and thoracic regions of the back, and as a preventive exercise for players who, because of their sport or playing style, frequently use rotation, hyperextension, or bending in the upper body.

Cobra Position

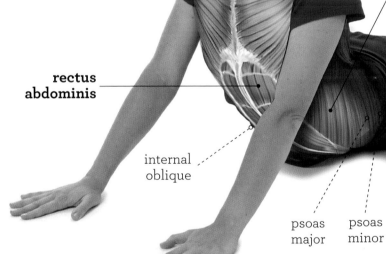

Starting Position

START

Lie face down, or in a prone position. Place your palms on the floor slightly to the side and ahead of your shoulders so that your elbows are bent and your forearms contact the floor. Gently straighten your elbows and raise your head and the upper part of your torso from the floor.

TECHNIQUE

Keep straightening your elbows slowly as if you were pushing against the floor. This will gradually move your chest away from your hands and extend your upper body. Your abdominal muscles will stretch, creating a sensation of tension that is easy to feel at the end of the motion; hold that position for a few seconds.

external oblique

rectus abdominis

internal oblique

psoas major

psoas minor

Keep your hips in contact with the floor.

	TENNIS	PADDLE.	SQUASH	FRONT.	BADMIN.
	✔			✔	✔

LEVEL	SETS	DURATION
BEGINNER	2	20 s
INTERMEDIATE	2	25 s
ADVANCED	2	30 s

CAUTION

Try to keep your hips in contact with the floor, or very close to it. If they rise from the floor the stretch will lose its effectiveness, so there will be no point in prolonging the movement.

INDICATION

For players who do sudden, powerful abdominal contractions, such as serves in tennis, high shots in badminton, or forehand shots in frontenis, since this exercise helps condition the abdominal muscles and protects them from injuries.

Upper-Body Extension on Fitness Ball

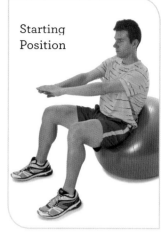

Starting Position

START
In order to do this stretch you will need a fitness ball or similar item, such as a bosu ball or a stability ball. Sit down on one side of the fitness ball, with both feet touching the floor and separated from one another for added stability. Put your hands together and straighten your elbows so that your arms and chest form an isosceles triangle with the most acute angle facing forward.

TECHNIQUE
Using shoulder antepulsion, raise your hands and make an arc so that they move overhead. From this point on, start to lean your upper body to the rear until your back rests on the fitness ball. Extend your spine so that your back conforms to the curvature of the fitness ball; this will stretch your abdominal muscles.

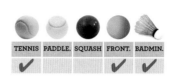

TENNIS	PADDLE.	SQUASH	FRONT.	BADMIN.
✔			✔	✔

LEVEL	SETS	DURATION
BEGINNER	2	20 s
INTERMEDIATE	2	25 s
ADVANCED	2	30 s

rectus abdominis

external oblique

internal oblique

Extend your spine so that it conforms to the curvature of the fitness ball.

CAUTION
Even though the fitness ball is a tremendously useful tool, it can be very unsteady, so you will need to start from a solid position and to do the exercise very deliberately, making sure to keep your balance throughout.

INDICATION
For athletes who make high, powerful shots, such as a tennis serve or an overhead because of the tension that is applied to the anterior muscle chain, including the abdominal muscles. Also for players of badminton and frontenis because of the many high and/or powerful shots that work the abdominal muscles for stability and performance of the technical move.

Upper-Body Rotation with Racket

Starting Position

Focus the movement on your upper body.

quadratus lumborum

external oblique
internal oblique

TENNIS	PADDLE.	SQUASH	FRONT.	BADMIN.
✔		✔		✔

LEVEL	SETS	DURATION
BEGINNER	2	15 s
INTERMEDIATE	2	20 s
ADVANCED	3	20 s

START

Stand and hold the racket with both hands so that the backs of your hands face upward and your thumbs are together. Keep both elbows straight and rotate your upper body slightly to the side where the head of the racket is located. Your companion should stand on the side that you are facing and slightly behind you, holding the frame of the racket on both sides.

TECHNIQUE

Your companion should slowly pull rearward on the racket, forcing you to rotate your upper body to keep holding the grip with both hands. Keep your feet in place, with your toes pointing forward as the upper part of your torso moves all the way to the side. This way, an imaginary line between your shoulders will be perpendicular to the same imaginary line drawn between your feet.

CAUTION

Remember that your hips need to stay in alignment with your feet, and the upper-body rotation should come solely from the torso, from your hips up. If the movement included your hips and legs, the effectiveness of the stretch would be greatly reduced.

INDICATION

For players whose disciplines require lots of upper-body rotation, including overheads, forehand shots, and backhand shots, either because of the force required to drive the ball, as in tennis and frontenis, or because of many high shots, as in badminton.

Upper-Body Rotation with Support

START

Stand in front of a vertical support that you can hang onto, maybe a pole, a trellis, a tree, or even a door frame. Hold onto the solid support with both hands, keeping your elbows straight and your upper body perpendicular to the floor. Your shoulders, hips, and feet should all be aligned with one another.

TECHNIQUE

Move your feet from their original position so that an imaginary line between them is perpendicular to a similar imaginary line drawn between your shoulders. The farther your feet rotate from their original position, the more intense the exercise. For maximum effectiveness, move your hips along with your feet.

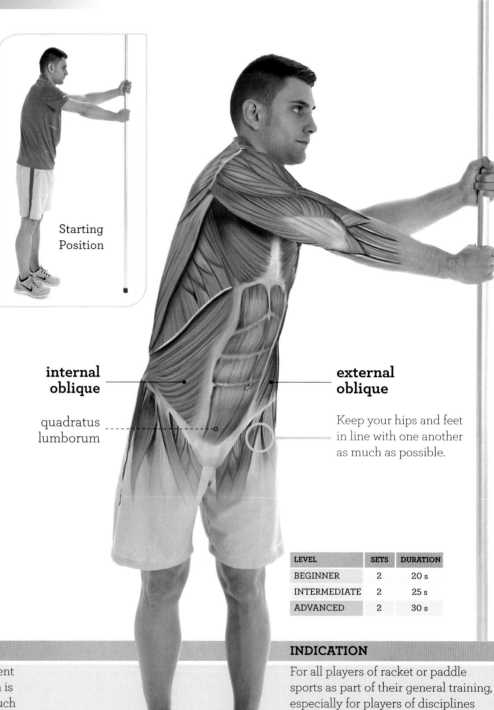

Starting Position

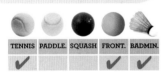

TENNIS	PADDLE.	SQUASH	FRONT.	BADMIN.
✔			✔	✔

internal oblique

quadratus lumborum

external oblique

Keep your hips and feet in line with one another as much as possible.

LEVEL	SETS	DURATION
BEGINNER	2	20 s
INTERMEDIATE	2	25 s
ADVANCED	2	30 s

CAUTION

Your hips need to stay in alignment with your feet so that the rotation is limited to your upper body as much as possible, in order to maximize the effectiveness of the stretch. So focus on the movement between your hips and shoulders, and use your feet only as a point of reference.

INDICATION

For all players of racket or paddle sports as part of their general training, especially for players of disciplines that require high and/or very powerful shots that involve the upper body as part of a kinetic chain, particularly in making shots.

Prone Upper-Body Rotation

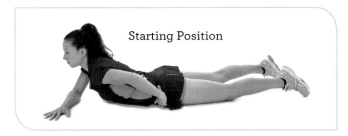

Starting Position

LEVEL	SETS	DURATION
BEGINNER	2	15 s
INTERMEDIATE	2	20 s
ADVANCED	2	25 s

TENNIS PADDLE. SQUASH FRONT. BADMIN.
✔   ✔   ✔

START

Lie face down, holding yourself up on one hand and forearm; look to the front and raise your chest from the floor. Place your free hand on your hip. Rest your thighs on the floor; keep your knees straight, with your toes touching the floor.

TECHNIQUE

Raise the shoulder opposite your support arm; this will cause extension and rotation in your upper body. Your abdomen will come off the floor as the stretch progresses, especially on the side of the higher shoulder. At the same time, use the hand on your hip to push it toward the floor; you soon will feel the tension from the stretch in both your abdomen and your lumbar region.

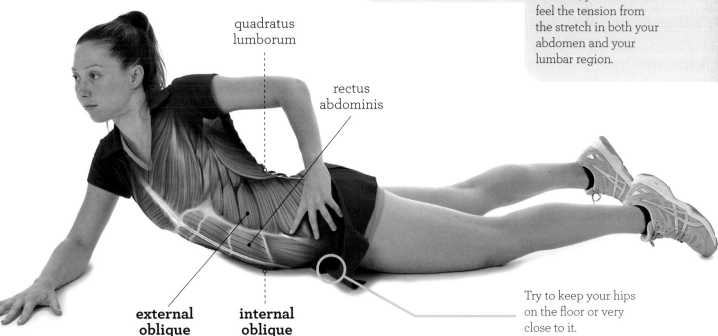

quadratus lumborum

rectus abdominis

external oblique

internal oblique

Try to keep your hips on the floor or very close to it.

CAUTION

Keep your hips in contact with or very close to the floor, limiting the extension and rotation movement to the area between your hips and shoulders. This will provide maximum efficiency in the stretch as well as spare you unnecessary movement and effort.

INDICATION

For athletes whose activity requires making powerful shots using the upper body as part of the kinetic chain, as in tennis and frontenis, or for others such as badminton players, who make lots of high shots that involve the muscles of the anterior chain, and more specifically the abdominal muscles.

SHOULDER AND CHEST STRETCHES

The importance of the shoulder in racket and paddle sports is clear. The variety of shoulder movements makes it possible to perform many types of shots, varying their height, trajectory, effect, power, and more. This great variety of movements certainly involves the action of many muscles that are responsible for the flexion, extension, abduction, adduction, internal and external rotation of this joint, in addition to many possible combinations of moves. Some of the most powerful muscles that act on the shoulder, such as the pectoralis major, the deltoids, and the latissimus dorsi, require adequate flexibility to allow broad movements along with fluid, efficient technique in the shots. Other muscles of smaller size and greater delicacy, such as the teres minor, the infraspinatus, and the subscapularis, can easily become strained with movements that require shoulder rotation, such as lift shots and slices, so they need to be strengthened and stretched for better performance and recovery.

PECTORALIS MAJOR

This powerful muscle has three different sections, much like the deltoid; however, because of their arrangement, they all serve fairly similar functions. The three of them share an insertion located at the crest of the greater tuberculum of the humerus.

Clavicular or Upper Portion: This part originates at the middle half of the clavicle; its main functions are adduction and flexion or antepulsion of the shoulder.

Sternocostal or Medial Portion: This part originates at the sternum and the costal cartilage of ribs 1 through 7. Its main function is shoulder adduction, especially horizontally, although it also contributes to retropulsion.

Abdominal or Lower Portion: This part originates at the aponeurosis of the external oblique; its main function is shoulder adduction, but it is also used to lower the arm from a raised position.

It is important to point out that even though all three parts are used in shoulder adduction, the degree of their involvement depends on the angle of flexion.

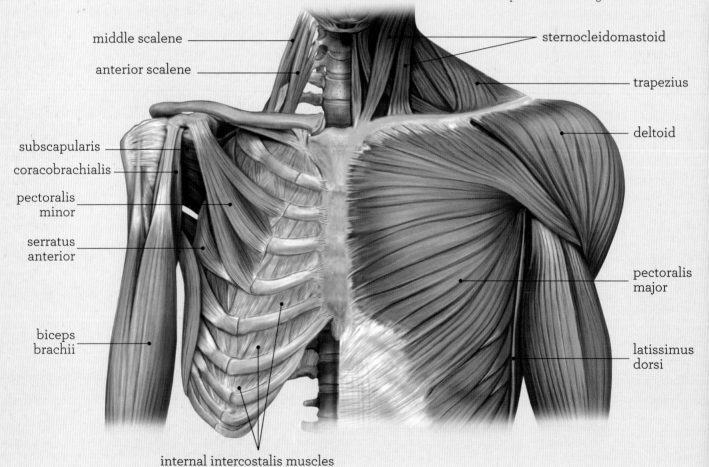

middle scalene

anterior scalene

sternocleidomastoid

trapezius

deltoid

subscapularis

coracobrachialis

pectoralis minor

serratus anterior

pectoralis major

biceps brachii

latissimus dorsi

internal intercostalis muscles

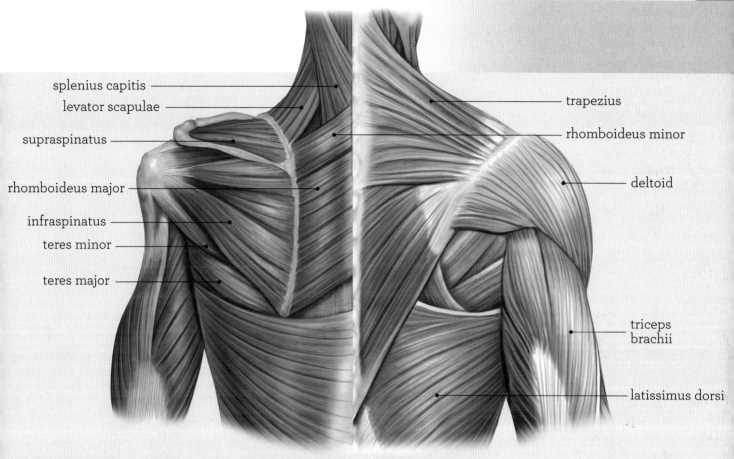

splenius capitis

levator scapulae

supraspinatus

rhomboideus major

infraspinatus

teres minor

teres major

trapezius

rhomboideus minor

deltoid

triceps brachii

latissimus dorsi

LATISSIMUS DORSI

This muscle originates at the spiny apophyses of vertebrae T7 to L5, the rear of the sacral bone, and the iliac crest. The insertion is at the crest of the lesser tuberculum of the humerus. The main function of this powerful muscle is shoulder adduction, but it is also used for internal rotation and retropulsion.

TERES MAJOR

This muscle originates at the lower angle of the scapula, and it inserts at the minor tuberculum of the humerus. Its main function is internal rotation of the shoulder, and to a lesser degree it contributes to adduction and retropulsion.

TERES MINOR

This muscle originates at the lateral edge of the scapula, and it inserts at the greater tuberculum of the humerus. Its main function is external rotation of the shoulder.

DELTOID

This muscle has three parts that are easy to identify; we know them according to the different functions that each one performs. All of them insert at the deltoid tuberosity of the humerus.

Clavicular or Anterior Part: This muscle originates at the distal third of the clavicle. Its main function is flexion or antepulsion of the shoulder, although it also participates in internal rotation and adduction.

Acromial or Middle Part: This muscle originates at the acromion, and its function is shoulder abduction.

Spiny or Posterior Part: This muscle originates at the spine of the scapula, and its main function is extension or retropulsion of the shoulder, although it also participates in external rotation and adduction.

INFRASPINATUS

This muscle originates at the infraspinous fossa of the scapula, and it inserts at the greater tuberculum of the humerus. Its function is external rotation of the shoulder.

SUBSCAPULARIS

This muscle originates at the subscapular fossa, and it inserts at the minor tuberculum of the humerus. Its function is internal rotation of the shoulder.

SERRATUS ANTERIOR

This muscle originates at ribs 1 through 9 and inserts at the medial edge of the scapula. Its upper part contributes to lowering the arm from a raised position; the central part causes abduction of the scapula; and the lower part rotates the scapula by moving its lower angle away from the spine.

Retropulsion with Racket

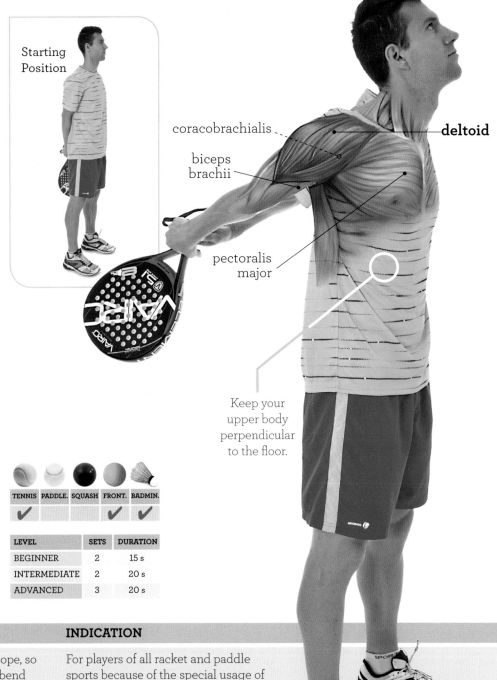

Starting Position

coracobrachialis · · · · · ·   **deltoid**

biceps
brachii

pectoralis
major

Keep your
upper body
perpendicular
to the floor.

START
Stand with your feet shoulder width apart and your upper body erect. Hold the paddle or racket behind your back with both hands on the grip. Your arms should remain relaxed, with your elbows straight so that the head of the paddle or racket points toward the floor.

TECHNIQUE
Using retropulsion of the shoulders, try to raise the paddle behind your body as far as possible, always keeping your upper body perpendicular to the floor and both hands on the grip. Even though this is an active stretch and the muscle tension you will experience is not the greatest, you may feel it in the front of your shoulder.

TENNIS	PADDLE.	SQUASH	FRONT.	BADMIN.
✔			✔	✔

LEVEL	SETS	DURATION
BEGINNER	2	15 s
INTERMEDIATE	2	20 s
ADVANCED	3	20 s

CAUTION
The movement is limited in scope, so there is a general tendency to bend your upper body or lean forward so that your hands, or in this case the paddle, goes higher. Avoid this error, for it contributes nothing to the stretch and it imposes unnecessary work on the back muscles.

INDICATION
For players of all racket and paddle sports because of the special usage of the shoulder joint and muscles in all disciplines, and especially for those who make high and/or powerful shots, such as tennis serves and overheads, as in tennis, frontenis, and badminton.

Double Rear Pull with Racket

pectoralis major

supraspinatus

deltoid

Straighten
your elbows
to increase
the tension in
your deltoids.

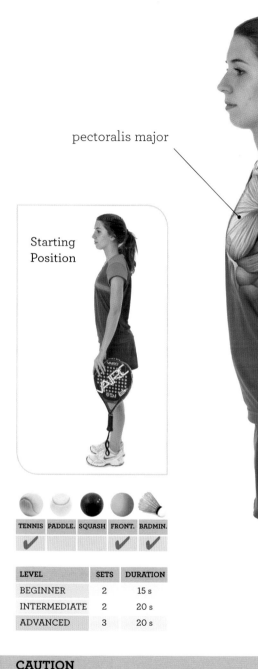

Starting
Position

TENNIS	PADDLE.	SQUASH	FRONT.	BADMIN.
✔			✔	✔

LEVEL	SETS	DURATION
BEGINNER	2	15 s
INTERMEDIATE	2	20 s
ADVANCED	3	20 s

START
Stand with your upper
body perpendicular to the
floor and hold the paddle
or racket by the side of
the frame. You can also
use a different item of
similar width, such as a
book, a Frisbee, or even
a ball. Keep your arms
relaxed and your elbows
straight.

TECHNIQUE
Hold the paddle
behind your back while
maintaining your original
grip on the side of
the head. Hold
the opposite
side of the
paddle
head with
your other
hand so
that your
forearms
are crossed
behind your
back. Then
try to straighten
your elbows as much as
possible, contract your
back muscles, and expand
your chest without
changing any of the
support points. You will
feel the muscle tension
in the front and middle
areas of your shoulders.

CAUTION
This stretch involves no particular risk, but
considering the intense work required of the
shoulders of participants in paddle and racket
sports and the many injuries they
incur, it's a good idea to pay attention
to the sensations you feel and stop
the exercise if you experience
pain in either shoulder during the
performance of the stretch.

INDICATION
For all players of paddle
or racket sports because
of the special use of the
shoulders in all disciplines,
and particularly if they feel
abnormal muscle tension
or, as with tennis and
badminton, they make high
and/or powerful shots.

Unilateral Retropulsion with Support

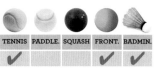

	TENNIS	PADDLE.	SQUASH	FRONT.	BADMIN.
	✓			✓	✓

LEVEL	SETS	DURATION
BEGINNER	2	20 s
INTERMEDIATE	2	25 s
ADVANCED	2	30 s

START

Stand next to a support such as a stool or a high chair. If you are at a court you can use the net or one of the posts that hold it up. Place the knuckles or the back of your hand on the support so that the palm faces rearward. Move one foot a long step ahead of the support and slightly bend both knees.

TECHNIQUE

By bending both knees, lower your upper body while keeping it perpendicular to the floor. As your center of gravity lowers, your hand should remain resting on the original support with your elbow straight so that you experience retropulsion in your shoulder, and thus the stretch in the front part of your deltoid.

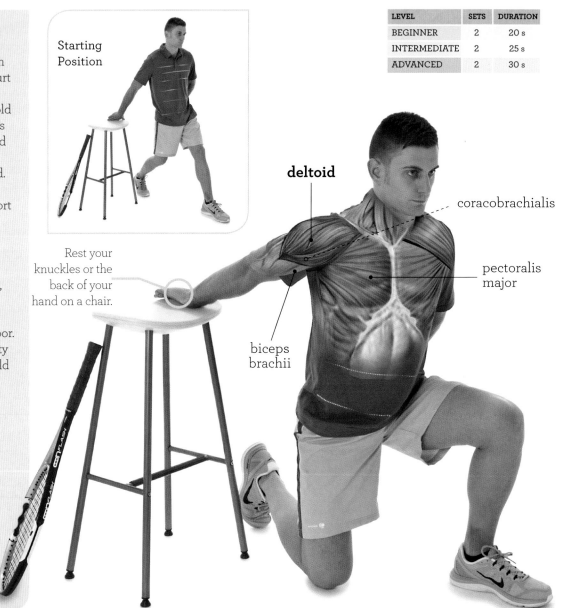

Starting Position

Rest your knuckles or the back of your hand on a chair.

deltoid

coracobrachialis

pectoralis major

biceps brachii

CAUTION

As your center of gravity moves downward, your upper body should remain perpendicular to the floor. Bending or leaning forward will not provide any advantage, even if that allows you to lower your center of gravity a little farther.

INDICATION

For all players of paddle and racket sports because of the involvement of the shoulder in all disciplines, and especially for those who feel strain in the shoulder muscles or who regularly make high and/or powerful shots, as it commonly happens in tennis, badminton, and frontenis.

Behind with Arm in Front

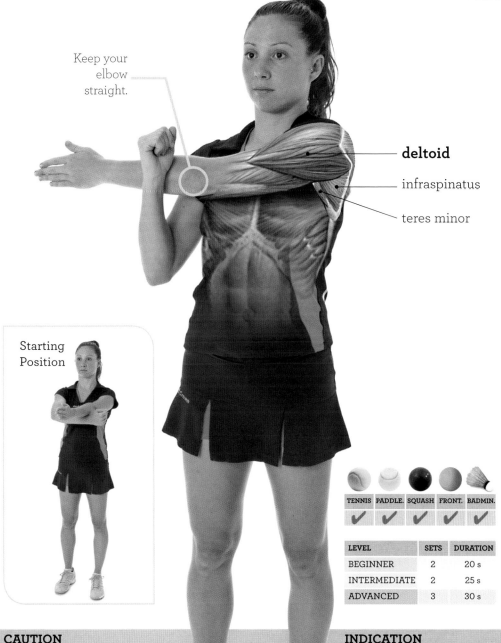

Keep your elbow straight.

deltoid

infraspinatus

teres minor

Starting Position

START
Stand and raise one arm via shoulder antepulsion to a 90° angle with your upper body. Your elbow should remain straight with your hand pointing straight ahead. Place your free hand behind the raised elbow so that your wrist contacts it.

TECHNIQUE
Bend the elbow on your support arm so that your wrist pulls on the opposite arm and brings it to your chest via frontal adduction of the shoulder. The elbow of the arm being stretched should remain totally straight. As your arm approaches your chest, you will feel the muscle tension from the stretch on the back part of your shoulder.

TENNIS	PADDLE.	SQUASH	FRONT.	BADMIN.
✓	✓	✓	✓	✓

LEVEL	SETS	DURATION
BEGINNER	2	20 s
INTERMEDIATE	2	25 s
ADVANCED	3	30 s

CAUTION
It is important for your elbow on the side being stretched to remain straight during the entire exercise to achieve the greatest efficiency. If you find this difficult, you can pull on your arm just above the elbow; in this case, the straightness of your elbow will not be important.

INDICATION
For all players of paddle and racket sports, especially those who make high shots or suffer discomfort in the rotator cuff, or who have experienced it in the past; also for players who wish to avoid this type of shoulder problem, which is very common especially among tennis players.

Front Elbow Pull

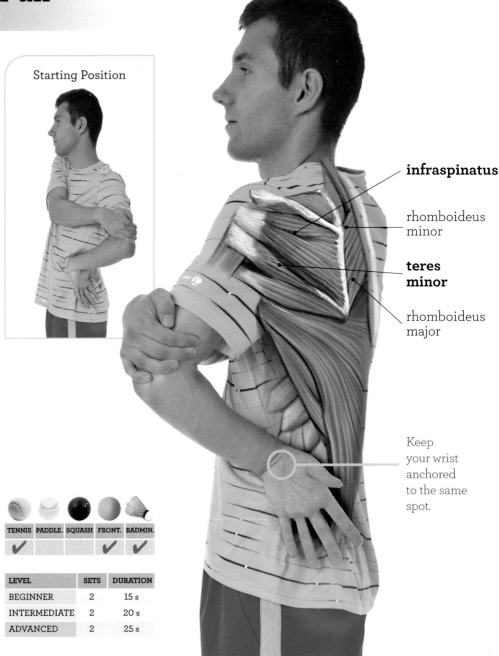

Starting Position

infraspinatus

rhomboideus minor

teres minor

rhomboideus major

Keep your wrist anchored to the same spot.

START
Stand with one hand on your waist. You can rest your wrist or the palm of your hand, so that one of your arms sticks out to the side. With your free hand, grasp the opposite elbow. You can hold the elbow or slightly above it, but you must grip firmly to perform the subsequent pull.

TECHNIQUE
Pull on the elbow so that it moves forward and toward the center, pivoting at the shoulder and the wrist resting on your waist; that anchor point should not move from its original position. You should pull gently for a short distance; you will soon feel the tension from the stretch in the rear of your shoulder.

TENNIS	PADDLE.	SQUASH	FRONT.	BADMIN.
✔			✔	✔

LEVEL	SETS	DURATION
BEGINNER	2	15 s
INTERMEDIATE	2	20 s
ADVANCED	2	25 s

CAUTION
This exercise stretches the external rotators of the shoulder; these muscles are not particularly robust, so the stretch should be done slowly and without exerting great force in the pull, in order to avoid hurting them or producing more stress in the area than you would experience in play.

INDICATION
For all players of racket and paddle sports because of the work that the external rotator muscles of the shoulder do in setting up for a forehand shot and a one-handed backhand. It is highly recommended for badminton and tennis players because of the frequent high shots that involve flexion and abduction of the shoulder above 90°, which can affect the rotator cuff.

TENNIS	PADDLE.	SQUASH	FRONT.	BADMIN.
✔			✔	✔

LEVEL	SETS	DURATION
BEGINNER	2	15 s
INTERMEDIATE	2	20 s
ADVANCED	2	25 s

Inverted Crank Position

supraspinatus

Rock the shaft of the racket on the rear of your shoulder.

infraspinatus

teres minor

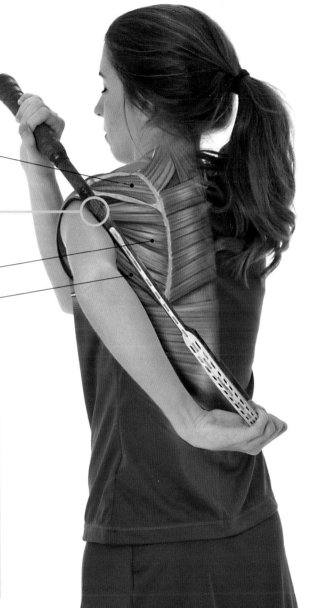

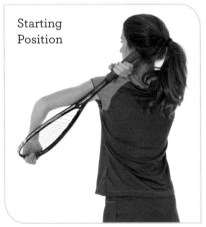

Starting Position

START
Stand and hold a racket, a walking stick, or similar item by the grip. Place the racket behind the opposite shoulder so that the head of the racket points downward. Use your free hand to hold the top of the frame of the racket head so that your forearm is in front of the strings and the palm of your hand faces rearward.

TECHNIQUE
Pull on the grip of the racket without letting go with the hand holding the frame, so that the shaft rocks on the back of your shoulder. This movement will produce internal rotation of the shoulder, and thus a stretch in the external rotator muscles; you will feel the muscle tension in the rear of your shoulder.

CAUTION
Do this stretch slowly and without much force as you pull on the grip; this will avoid discomfort in the muscles being stretched. Do not use too much pressure as the shaft of the racket contacts your shoulder, and before starting the movement, be sure that the racket is stable and you have a solid grip on it.

INDICATION
For practically all players of racket and paddle sports because of the work that these muscles perform in many common shots; especially for players whose disciplines involve high shots in which the antepulsion or abduction of the shoulder exceeds 90°, because of the greater risk of affecting the rotator cuff.

Support with Elbow Pivot

subscapularis

teres major

Keep your upper arm in contact with your body.

START

Stand next to some solid vertical object that you can use for support; this can be a column, a corner, a door frame, or anything else that will serve as a support. Advance the foot that is farther away from the support and bend the elbow that is closer to it to about 90°. Rest the bent elbow on your waist, and use the same hand to grasp the support, which should be slightly ahead of your body.

TECHNIQUE

Take a small step ahead with your rear foot so that it is in front of the other one. This will move your body ahead. Maintain your grasp on the solid support and keep your elbow on your hip so that it acts as a pivot. As your position moves forward with respect to the vertical support your shoulder will rotate outward, thereby stretching some of your internal rotators.

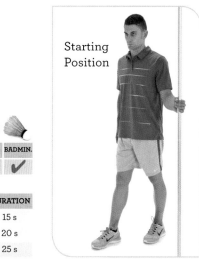

Starting Position

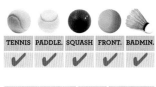

TENNIS	PADDLE.	SQUASH	FRONT.	BADMIN.
✔	✔	✔	✔	✔

LEVEL	SETS	DURATION
BEGINNER	2	15 s
INTERMEDIATE	2	20 s
ADVANCED	2	25 s

CAUTION

As with all exercises that involve the shoulder joint, be prudent and do the exercises slowly and gradually, proceeding with caution if you feel any pain or discomfort beyond the discomfort from the stretch.

INDICATION

For all athletes in paddle and racket sports because of the strenuous task that the internal rotator muscles perform in the forehand, the overhead, and the serve in tennis, among other movements; also for people who experience muscle discomfort, problems with the rotator muscles, or instability in the shoulder. In the latter case, they should combine this stretch with strengthening exercises for these muscles.

Crank Position

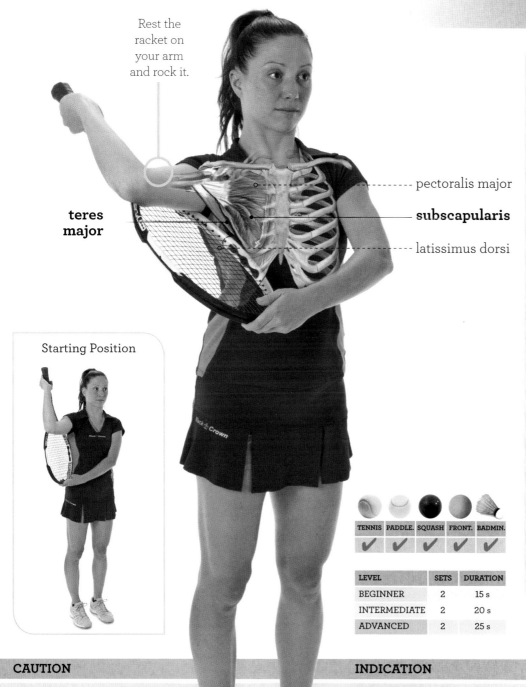

Rest the racket on your arm and rock it.

teres major

pectoralis major

subscapularis

latissimus dorsi

Starting Position

START
In a standing position, hold your racket or something similar, such as a walking stick or a rod, by the grip. Perform shoulder abduction and bend your elbow to 90° in both cases, and lower the head of the racket behind your arm. Using the fingertips of your free hand, grasp the top of the frame.

TECHNIQUE
Pull on the handle of the racket with your lower hand, while maintaining the shoulder abduction at a 90° angle. The throat of the racket will rock on your arm, causing the raised forearm and hand to incline rearward and produce the external rotation of the shoulder. You probably will feel the tension from the stretch below your scapula.

TENNIS	PADDLE.	SQUASH	FRONT.	BADMIN.
✔	✔	✔	✔	✔

LEVEL	SETS	DURATION
BEGINNER	2	15 s
INTERMEDIATE	2	20 s
ADVANCED	2	25 s

CAUTION
Use gentle force on the frame of the racket and perform the movement slowly to protect the integrity of the muscles being stretched and the shoulder joint; this stretch affects a relatively sensitive area.

INDICATION
For athletes who have experienced muscle discomfort in the shoulder; it is preferable to do this stretch in combination with muscle strengthening exercises. Also for players of racket or paddle sports because of the special use of the internal rotator muscles of the shoulder in the forehand, overhead, and serve in tennis, among others.

Assisted Seated Pull

START

You will need the help of an assistant for this exercise. Sit down with your back perpendicular to the floor, place your hands behind your neck, and lock your fingers together. Your helper should place the side of one leg against your back to serve as a rest, and place his hands on the inside of your elbows.

TECHNIQUE

Your helper should slowly pull your elbows rearward, while avoiding leaning to the rear with his leg. Your elbows will move toward the rear from their original position due to the horizontal abduction of the shoulder; this will produce a stretch mainly in the pectoralis major. You will clearly feel muscle tension in your chest as your helper applies more force in pulling your elbows back.

Starting Position

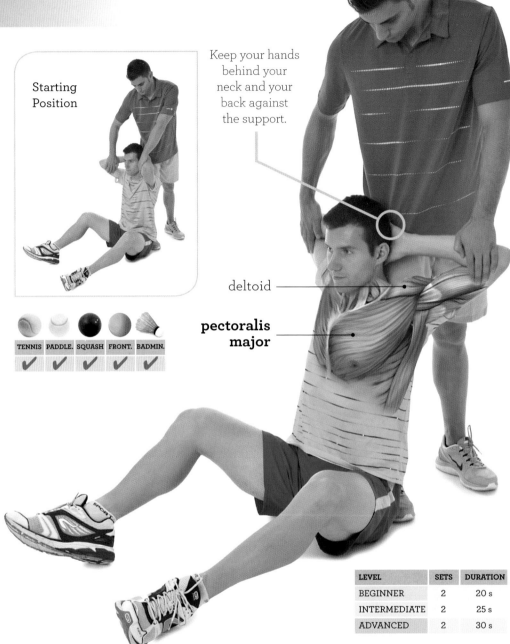

Keep your hands behind your neck and your back against the support.

deltoid

pectoralis major

TENNIS	PADDLE.	SQUASH	FRONT.	BADMIN.
✓	✓	✓	✓	✓

LEVEL	SETS	DURATION
BEGINNER	2	20 s
INTERMEDIATE	2	25 s
ADVANCED	2	30 s

CAUTION

As with all assisted stretches, especially with the help of a non-professional, communication must be constant so you don't exceed the range of motion or the proper level of muscle tension, or damage the joint and the surrounding structures.

INDICATION

For all players of racket and paddle sports because of the involvement of the pectoralis major in the forehand shot in all its variants, and in preparation for the one-handed backhand, especially if they feel unaccustomed muscle tension in the pectoralis major.

Vertical Support on One Side

	TENNIS	PADDLE.	SQUASH	FRONT.	BADMIN.
	✔	✔	✔	✔	✔

LEVEL	SETS	DURATION
BEGINNER	2	20 s
INTERMEDIATE	2	25 s
ADVANCED	2	30 s

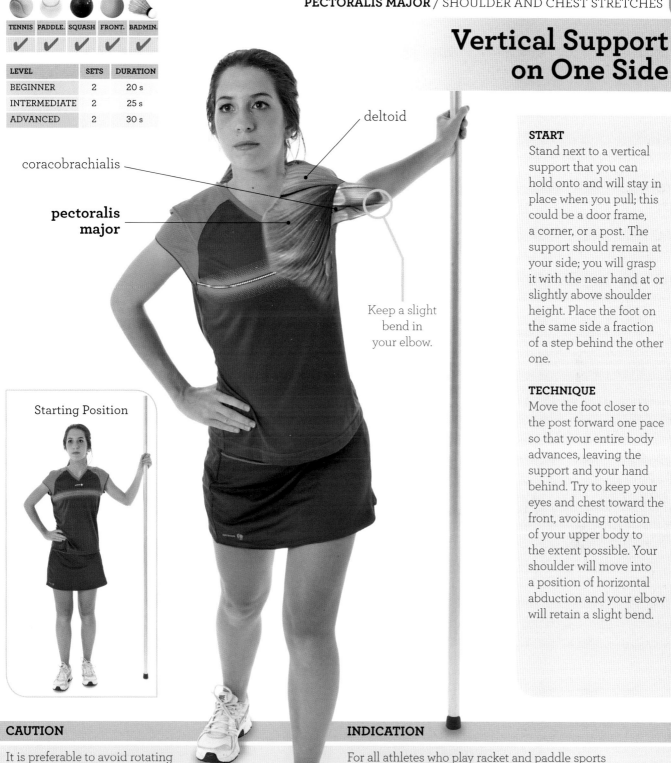

coracobrachialis

pectoralis major

deltoid

Keep a slight bend in your elbow.

Starting Position

START
Stand next to a vertical support that you can hold onto and will stay in place when you pull; this could be a door frame, a corner, or a post. The support should remain at your side; you will grasp it with the near hand at or slightly above shoulder height. Place the foot on the same side a fraction of a step behind the other one.

TECHNIQUE
Move the foot closer to the post forward one pace so that your entire body advances, leaving the support and your hand behind. Try to keep your eyes and chest toward the front, avoiding rotation of your upper body to the extent possible. Your shoulder will move into a position of horizontal abduction and your elbow will retain a slight bend.

CAUTION
It is preferable to avoid rotating your upper body, and to keep a slight bend in your elbow to focus the stretch on the pectoral and avoid splitting the stretch between the pectoral and the flexor muscles of the elbow. This will optimize the results from the exercise.

INDICATION
For all athletes who play racket and paddle sports because of the high demands on the muscles that perform frontal adduction in the forehand shot and the setup for the one-handed backhand, among others. Also for people who feel muscle discomfort in the pectoralis major, or who wish to expand the range of certain shoulder movements.

Support with Elbow Bend

START

Stand next to a sturdy vertical support such as a post or a door frame. With the support beside you, place the foot nearer to it one step behind the other one. Perform the abduction and external rotation of the shoulder and bend your elbow so that both remain at 90°, and rest your hand and forearm on the support. The palm of your hand will face forward with your fingers pointing up.

TECHNIQUE

Move the rear foot forward one step, keeping the other one in place and moving your whole body ahead; this will produce the horizontal abduction of your shoulder. Your forearm and support hand will stay in the same place on the support, and the length of your pace will determine the intensity of the stretch.

Contact the vertical support with your hand and forearm.

pectoralis major

deltoid

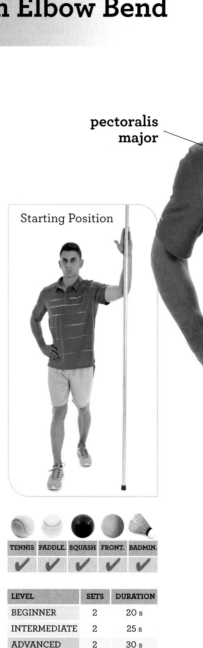

Starting Position

TENNIS	PADDLE.	SQUASH	FRONT.	BADMIN.
✔	✔	✔	✔	✔

LEVEL	SETS	DURATION
BEGINNER	2	20 s
INTERMEDIATE	2	25 s
ADVANCED	2	30 s

CAUTION

It is important to avoid rotating your upper body toward the support, since this maneuver would diminish the frontal abduction of the shoulder and thus reduce or eliminate the stretch in the pectoralis major. Also keep in mind that if you feel any pain in your shoulder, you should immediately reduce the intensity of the stretch.

INDICATION

For all players of racket and paddle sports because of the involvement of the pectoralis major in the various shots, and the improvement that keeping this muscle strong and flexible can bring to your playing, in terms of power and range of movement.

Support with Elbow Bend and Helper

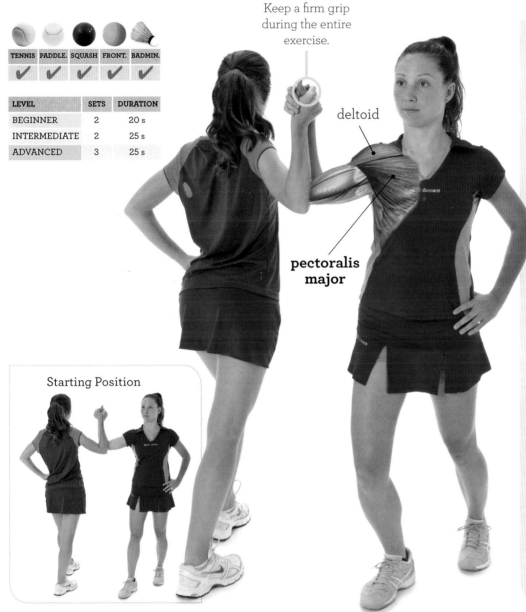

Keep a firm grip during the entire exercise.

deltoid

pectoralis major

	TENNIS	PADDLE.	SQUASH	FRONT.	BADMIN.
	✔	✔	✔	✔	✔

LEVEL	SETS	DURATION
BEGINNER	2	20 s
INTERMEDIATE	2	25 s
ADVANCED	3	25 s

Starting Position

START

To do this exercise you will need help from a friend, who will do the stretch at the same time. Stand beside one another, facing opposite directions, and hold hands so that your forearms contact one another and your fists point upward, almost as if you were arm wrestling. Keep one foot slightly ahead of the other.

TECHNIQUE

Move your upper body forward without moving your feet from their original anchor points; this will put you into a slight forward lean, as if you were pushing or pulling a heavy object. Keep firm contact between your hands and forearms; this will produce horizontal abduction of the shoulder and the attendant stretch in the pectoralis major.

CAUTION

Look straight ahead and avoid rotating your upper body to maximize the effect of the stretch and concentrate it in your pectoralis major. Rotating your upper body toward your helper will reduce the effectiveness of the stretch, and rotating it in the other direction could increase it; however, this will not be necessary unless the technique described is not sufficiently intense.

INDICATION

For all players of racket and paddle sports because of the involvement of the pectoralis major in many shots, and the noticeable improvement in playing that keeping this muscle as strong and flexible as possible so it can execute broader movements and more powerful shots, especially in the forehand.

Plank Position

START

Lie face down, or in a prone position. Contact the floor with the tips of your toes, your thighs, your elbows, and your forearms, and lift up your chest. Your upper body and legs should be in alignment, and the center of your back should be higher than your shoulders, so that your upper body is under tension, and slight to moderate effort is required to maintain the position.

TECHNIQUE

Slightly relax the upper part of your body to reduce the tension in the muscles of your scapular girdle so that your chest and abdomen move downward and the middle of your back descends to a point lower than your shoulder blades, which experience the adduction necessary for stretching the serratus anterior.

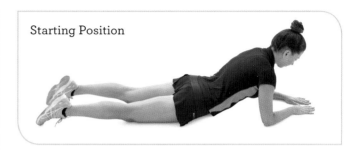

Starting Position

Lower the center of your back.

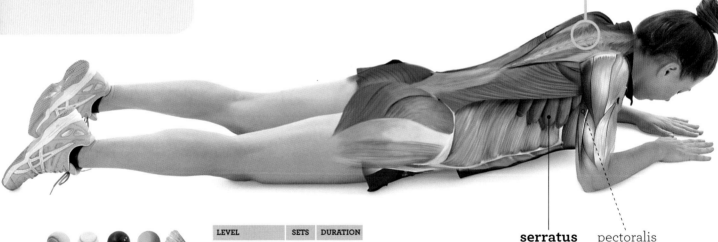

serratus anterior

pectoralis minor

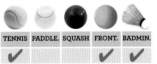

	TENNIS	PADDLE.	SQUASH	FRONT.	BADMIN.
	✔			✔	✔

LEVEL	SETS	DURATION
BEGINNER	2	15 s
INTERMEDIATE	2	20 s
ADVANCED	2	20 s

CAUTION

The serratus anterior helps secure the scapula to your thorax, so we must not overdo the stretches for this muscle, since they could affect the attachment function, especially if we recall that it is not particularly powerful, and that problems related to inadequate functioning, such as scapula alata or winged scapula, are fairly common.

INDICATION

For all players of racket or paddle sports, except those who have problems with the attachment of the scapula to the thorax, and particularly for players whose disciplines require many high shots, as in badminton.

Bilateral Pull with Helper

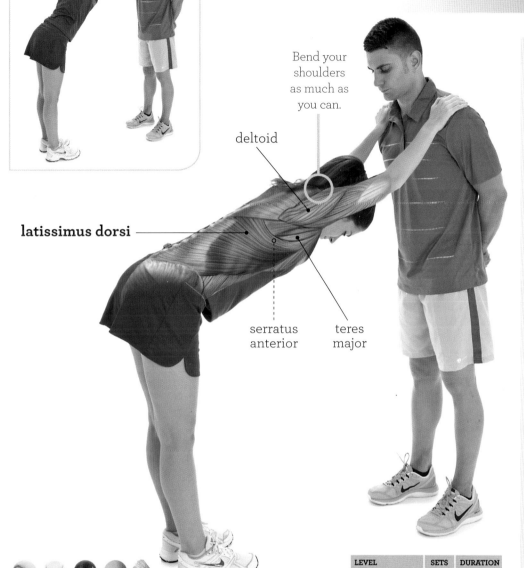

Starting Position

Bend your shoulders as much as you can.

deltoid

latissimus dorsi

serratus anterior

teres major

TENNIS	PADDLE.	SQUASH	FRONT.	BADMIN.
✔			✔	✔

START
Stand facing a helper, who will act as a support. You should be slightly more than one normal step apart from one another. Bend your upper body forward from the waist and rest your hands on your helper's shoulders, keeping your elbows almost totally straight.

TECHNIQUE
Lower your chest toward the floor by bending farther at the hips and without bending your upper body. Keep your hands on your friend's shoulders; this will limit your movement and force you to bend your shoulders significantly, which in turn will stretch your latissimus dorsi and other muscles.

LEVEL	SETS	DURATION
BEGINNER	2	20 s
INTERMEDIATE	2	25 s
ADVANCED	2	25 s

CAUTION
Avoid bending your upper body, and pay particular attention to how your shoulders feel: at the end of this movement they will be in maximum antepulsion, and subjecting them to tension may cause pain or instability. Oftentimes these signals are the prelude to an injury, so if they appear, you should immediately reduce the intensity of the stretch.

INDICATION
For athletes who feel tension or muscle pain in the area of the latissimus dorsi, especially if it appears while performing a serve, overhead, or high shots in tennis. Discomfort may arise in both the backswing and the advance because of the particular involvement of the latissimus dorsi in these movements, whether through contraction or stretching.

Side Lean with Elbow Pull

START

Stand with your upper body perpendicular to the floor. Raise your arms using antepulsion of the shoulders. Bend your elbows so that your forearms cross behind your head. Keep your feet far enough apart for stability even when you move slightly to one side of your center of gravity.

TECHNIQUE

Hold one elbow with the opposite hand and pull on it behind your head as you lean your upper body to the side by bending your spine. The combination of these two movements will produce the stretch in the latissimus dorsi, which you will feel in the side of your back. This is one of the most effective exercises for this area.

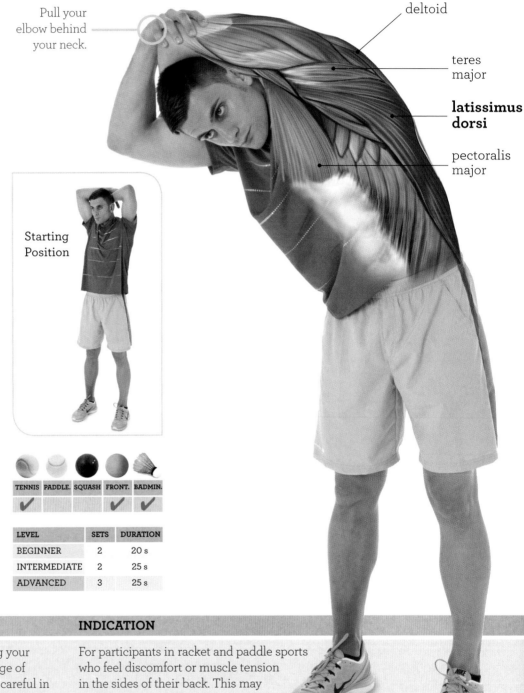

Pull your elbow behind your neck.

deltoid

teres major

latissimus dorsi

pectoralis major

Starting Position

TENNIS	PADDLE.	SQUASH	FRONT.	BADMIN.
✔		✔	✔	

LEVEL	SETS	DURATION
BEGINNER	2	20 s
INTERMEDIATE	2	25 s
ADVANCED	3	25 s

CAUTION

This exercise involves moving your shoulder to the limit of its range of movement, so you need to be careful in pulling, especially if you feel any pain in your joint. Also make sure you have a solid support base so you can keep your balance while doing this stretch.

INDICATION

For participants in racket and paddle sports who feel discomfort or muscle tension in the sides of their back. This may be due to repeated stretching and contraction, especially in the case of the latissimus dorsi and the teres major muscles in high shots such as overheads and serves in tennis; tennis and badminton players may be most affected by this.

Side Lean with Assisted Pull

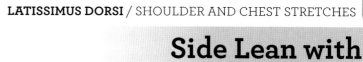

Starting Position

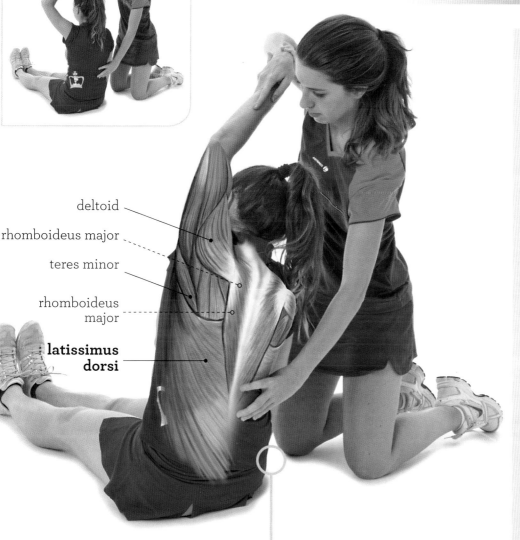

deltoid

rhomboideus major

teres minor

rhomboideus major

latissimus dorsi

Keep one hand on the floor to stabilize the position.

START

Sit down with your upper body perpendicular to the floor, your knees straight, and your thighs and feet together in front of you. Raise one hand and put the other one on the floor for support. Your helper will kneel next to your support hand, grasp your other wrist, and place the other hand near your waist to keep you from bending your upper body.

TECHNIQUE

Your helper should pull rearward and upward on your wrist so that your elbow is straight over your head. Your helper will push on your waist with the other hand to keep your whole body from leaning, so that your spine bends to the side. You will feel the muscle tension to the side of your spine, and it will be most intense in the area near your armpit.

TENNIS	PADDLE.	SQUASH	FRONT.	BADMIN.
✔			✔	✔

LEVEL	SETS	DURATION
BEGINNER	2	15 s
INTERMEDIATE	2	20 s
ADVANCED	3	20 s

CAUTION

Be sure to communicate effectively with your helper so you are not subjected to excessive force in the pull or the push. It is also helpful if you both have about the same reach so that the range of movement and the applied force are appropriate.

INDICATION

For tennis and badminton players because of the many high shots they make that require consecutive rapid, broad, and powerful stretching and contraction of the latissimus dorsi and other muscles; these moves can affect the integrity of these muscles, especially if they are not in the best condition.

ARM AND HAND STRETCHES

The movements of the elbow, the wrist, and the shoulder are mainly responsible for the various shots used in racket and paddle sports, so the muscles that move these joints deserve special care. Muscles like the biceps and triceps brachii are not commonly subject to strain since they are so powerful, but they need to be kept flexible so they can perform broad movements, especially in the case of the biceps brachii, which is in contraction when the player is in the ready position. The epicondylian and epitrochlear muscles may cause problems from overuse; this frequently happens in the racket sports with tennis elbow, which comes from repeated use of the backhand, and golfer's elbow, which, despite its name, also affects players of racket and paddle sports, mainly through the use of the topspin forehand shot. Also, gripping the racket involves continuous use of the flexor muscles of the fingers, so it is important to do exercises to improve their flexibility.

BICEPS BRACHII
The long head originates at the supraglenoid tubercle, and the short head at the coracoid apophysis of the scapula. Both heads join and insert at the radial tuberosity. Their main function is bending the elbow, but they also are used for supination, and they play a role in antepulsion of the shoulder.

TRICEPS BRACHII
The long head originates at the infraglenoid tubercle of the scapula; the medial head at the two distal thirds of the diaphysis of the humerus on its posterior face, and the lateral head at the proximal third of the diaphysis of the humerus, likewise at the posterior face. They all insert at the olecranon of the ulna. Their main function is straightening the elbow, with minor participation in shoulder retropulsion and adduction.

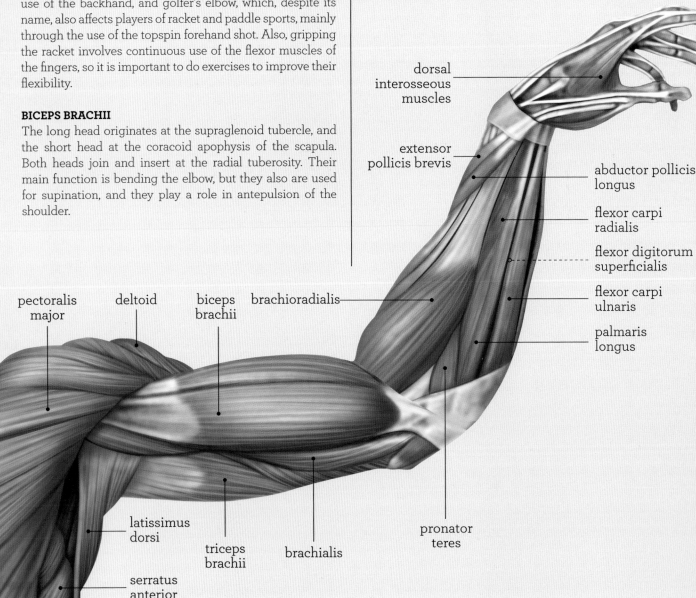

dorsal interosseous muscles

extensor pollicis brevis

abductor pollicis longus

flexor carpi radialis

flexor digitorum superficialis

flexor carpi ulnaris

palmaris longus

pectoralis major

deltoid

biceps brachii

brachioradialis

latissimus dorsi

triceps brachii

brachialis

pronator teres

serratus anterior

FLEXOR CARPI RADIALIS
This muscle originates at the medial epicondyle of the humerus or epitrochlea, and it inserts at the base of the second metacarpal. Its functions are flexion and abduction of the hand.

EXTENSOR CARPI RADIALIS
This muscle originates at the lateral epicondyle of the humerus, and it inserts at the base of the third metacarpal. Its main functions, which if shares with the long radial extensor of the wrist, are extension and abduction of the wrist, and it also participates slightly in bending the elbow.

EXTENSOR CARPI RADIALIS LONGUS
This muscle originates at the lateral supracondylar crest of the humerus, and it inserts at the base of the second metacarpal.

FLEXOR DIGITORUM SUPERFICIALIS
This muscle originates at the medial epicondyle of the humerus or epitrochlea, the coronoid apophysis of the ulna, and the anterior diaphysis of the radius, and it inserts at the second phalange of fingers two through five. Its functions are flexion of the wrist and fingers, except for the thumb.

FLEXOR POLLICIS BREVIS
This muscle originates at the flexor retinaculum and the capitate and trapezium bones, and it inserts at the base of the first proximal phalange. Its function is flexion in the metacarpophalangeal joint of the thumb.

FLEXOR POLLICIS LONGUS
This muscle originates at the anterior face of the radius and the interosseous membrane, and it inserts at the distal phalange. Its functions are flexion of the thumb in its carpometacarpal, metacarpophalangeal, and interphalangeal joints, plus flexion and abduction of the wrist.

EXTENSOR DIGITORUM
This muscle originates at the lateral epicondyle of the humerus, and it inserts at the phalanges of fingers two through five, through the dorsal aponeurotic expansion. Its main functions are extension of the wrist and fingers two through five in the metacarpophalangeal and interphalangeal joints.

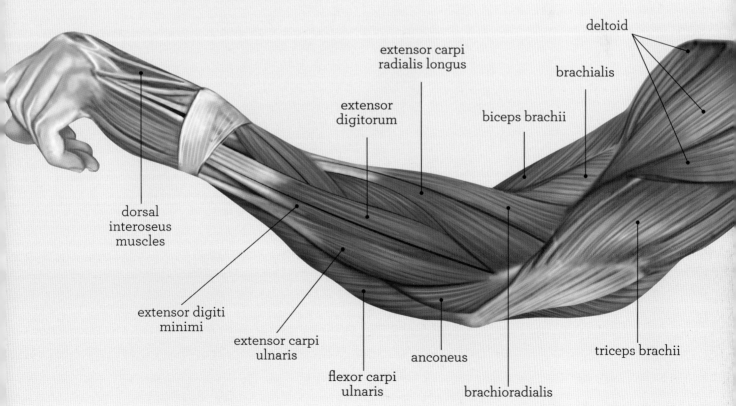

Pull from Rear

START

Stand near a vertical support that you can hold onto, such as a post or a door frame. Turn your back to it, with one foot ahead of the other; stand close enough so you can hold the support with one hand. You will have to place your hand in pronation, so that your thumb and the front of your elbow point downward.

TECHNIQUE

Bend both knees and lower your center of gravity while keeping your grip in the original position. As your center of gravity moves downward, your shoulder will move into extension; in combination with your elbow, this will cause a stretch in both heads of the biceps brachii.

Starting Position

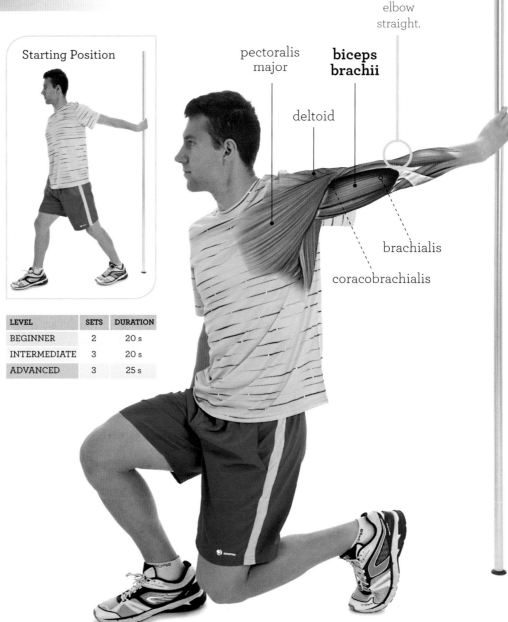

Keep your elbow straight.

pectoralis major

biceps brachii

deltoid

brachialis

coracobrachialis

LEVEL	SETS	DURATION
BEGINNER	2	20 s
INTERMEDIATE	3	20 s
ADVANCED	3	25 s

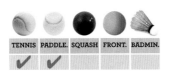

TENNIS	PADDLE.	SQUASH	FRONT.	BADMIN.
✔	✔			

CAUTION

Bend your knees slowly and control the lowering of your center of gravity and the speed of the stretch. Remember that the shoulder will reach a significant degree of extension, so you will have to pay attention to any pain in both the shoulder and the biceps brachii.

INDICATION

For players who feel discomfort in the front part of the shoulder, who have previously had tendonitis in the large head of the biceps brachii, or who frequently make shots that involve the simultaneous flexion of the shoulder and elbow, as in the case of the topspin forehand, especially if the end of the movement is high.

Assisted Retropulsion

deltoid

brachialis

coracobrachialis
pectoralis major

biceps brachii

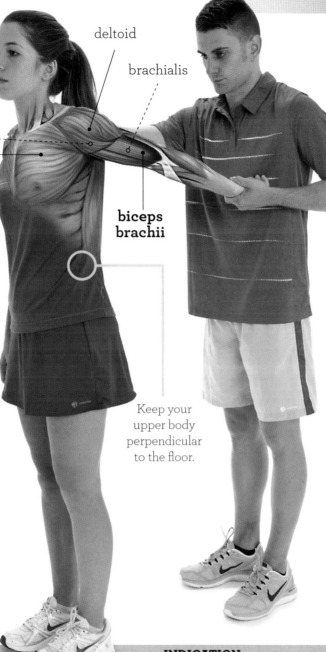

Keep your upper body perpendicular to the floor.

Starting Position

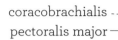

TENNIS	PADDLE.	SQUASH	FRONT.	BADMIN.
✔	✔			

LEVEL	SETS	DURATION
BEGINNER	2	20 s
INTERMEDIATE	3	20 s
ADVANCED	3	25 s

START

To do this exercise you will need the help of a friend, who will take a position about one step behind you. Both of you face the same direction. Your friend will place one hand on your shoulder, and the other hand will hold your opposite wrist; keep the elbow on this side straight.

TECHNIQUE

Your friend will pull your wrist upward, producing retropulsion in your shoulder. Your elbow should remain straight throughout the movement. If your friend turns your wrist toward the inside, producing pronation of your forearm, this will optimize the stretch, and you will feel it on the front of your arm.

CAUTION

This stretch involves no specific risk, but your helper needs to perform the movement slowly and be responsive to your instructions; constant communication will keep you from stretching too far or exposing yourself to any risk.

INDICATION

Particularly for players who have experienced discomfort in the front of the shoulder or arm, have had tendonitis in the large head of the biceps brachii, or who play hard and regularly use the topspin forehand shot, especially if the end of the movement is very high.

Seated Shoulder Extension

START

Sit down with your legs together and your knees straight. Place both hands behind your gluteal muscles and about shoulder width apart. Both hands should be in supination so that your fingers point rearward. Your elbows should be completely straight.

TECHNIQUE

Slide forward on your gluteal muscles while maintaining the initial support points for your hands and feet; this will cause your knees to bend and your shoulders to extend. Along with the extension in your elbows, this shoulder extension will produce the bilateral stretch in your biceps brachii.

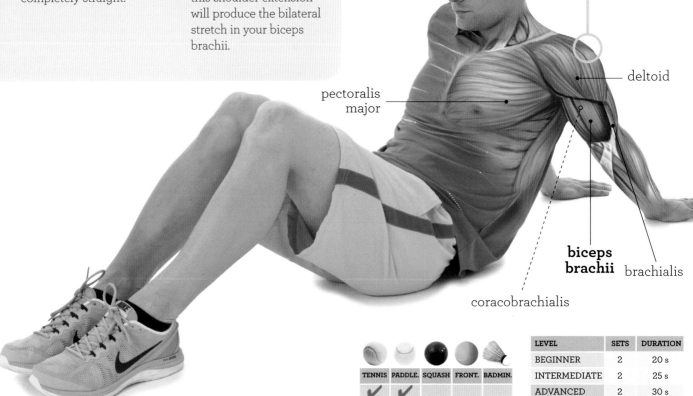

Keep your shoulders and elbows extended.

deltoid

pectoralis major

biceps brachii brachialis

coracobrachialis

	TENNIS	PADDLE.	SQUASH	FRONT.	BADMIN.
	✔	✔			

LEVEL	SETS	DURATION
BEGINNER	2	20 s
INTERMEDIATE	2	25 s
ADVANCED	2	30 s

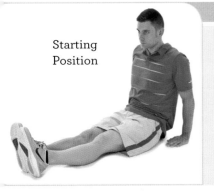

Starting Position

CAUTION

Pay attention to any signs of discomfort or pain in your shoulders, since they will be in maximum extension at the end of the movement; any minor extension could be counterproductive.

INDICATION

Especially for players who often use shots that combine flexion of the shoulder and elbow, such as the topspin forehand that is commonly used in tennis, paddleball, and to a lesser degree in other paddle or racket sports, because of their susceptibility to tendonitis in the long head of the biceps brachii.

Rear Elbow Pull

Keep your elbow
bent as you pull
it to the rear.

triceps brachii

deltoid

teres major

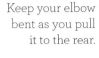

LEVEL	SETS	DURATION
BEGINNER	2	20 s
INTERMEDIATE	2	25 s
ADVANCED	3	25 s

latissimus
dorsi

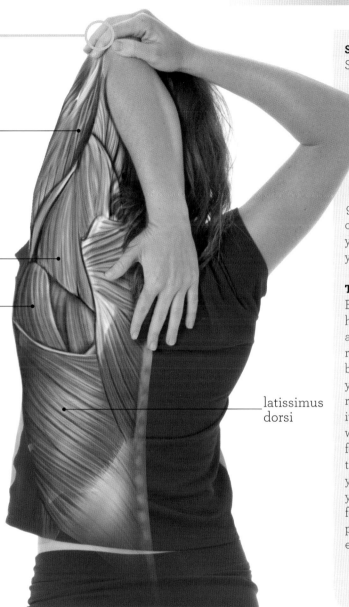

START
Stand with your upper
body perpendicular
to the floor and
your head inclined
slightly forward,
and raise one arm
so that it is in line
with your upper body.
Bend your elbow to
90° and hold it with the
opposite hand so that
your forearm is above
your head.

TECHNIQUE
Bend the elbow you are
holding as far as possible,
as if you were trying to
reach the middle of your
back with your hand; use
your other hand to pull it
rearward, trying to move
it behind your head. You
will quickly and clearly
feel the tension from
the stretch in the rear of
your arm. You can move
your head a little farther
forward to facilitate
performance of this
exercise.

Starting Position

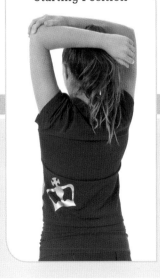

CAUTION
If you feel pain in your shoulder
that exceeds the discomfort from a
stretch, slightly reduce the intensity
of the exercise until it disappears.
It is always preferable to safeguard
the integrity of the joint.

INDICATION
For players who feel tension or
muscle discomfort in the rear of
the elbow; this may occur from
repeated use of the backhand
shot, especially with one hand,
if lots of force is used.

Rear Pull with Racket

START

You can use your racket or some other item of similar length that you can hold by both ends and pull on. Stand while holding the racket by the grip and place it behind your back so that the strings are behind your head. Use your free hand to hold the top of the frame so that your wrist is above your head.

TECHNIQUE

Using the hand that is holding the grip of the racket, pull it downward while maintaining your grip on the frame. This will produce a sharp bend in the elbow of the raised arm; your shoulder on the same side will accentuate the position of antepulsion, and this will stretch the triceps brachii. You will feel the tension in the back of the raised arm.

triceps brachii

Bend your shoulder and elbow as far as possible.

deltoid

teres major

latissimus dorsi

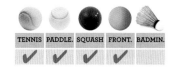

TENNIS	PADDLE.	SQUASH	FRONT.	BADMIN.
✔	✔	✔	✔	

LEVEL	SETS	DURATION
BEGINNER	2	20 s
INTERMEDIATE	2	25 s
ADVANCED	3	25 s

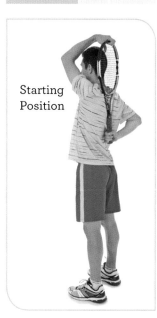

Starting Position

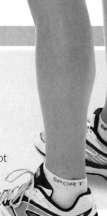

CAUTION

This stretch does not involve any notable risk. Merely try to keep your grip on the frame, which is precarious, as comfortable and solid as possible before starting to pull down on the grip; this will keep you from having to stop and reposition your fingers halfway through the exercise.

INDICATION

Especially for people who play hard, with powerful one-handed backhand shots, because of the sudden and simultaneous extension in the elbow and shoulder; in the medium and long term this can lead to muscle and tendon problems, especially in the long head of the triceps brachii if it is not trained properly.

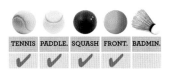

TENNIS	PADDLE.	SQUASH	FRONT.	BADMIN.
✓	✓	✓	✓	

LEVEL	SETS	DURATION
BEGINNER	2	20 s
INTERMEDIATE	2	25 s
ADVANCED	3	25 s

Bilateral Rear Pull

triceps brachii

deltoid

teres major

latissimus dorsi

Avoid hyperextension of your lumbar vertebrae.

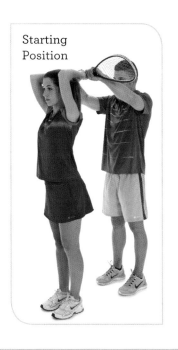

Starting Position

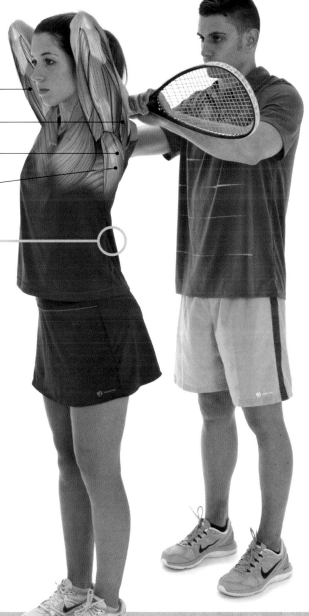

START

In order to do this exercise you will need your racket and the help of a friend. Stand and hold your racket with both hands on the grip and the shaft so that your palms face downward and your thumbs face each other. Raise your arms and bend your elbows to 90° so that your racket is behind your head. Your friend should take a position behind you and hold the racket with both hands next to yours.

TECHNIQUE

Your helper should pull the racket downward while keeping it parallel to the floor; your shoulders and elbows will bend as far as possible and symmetrically. Your arms will be at the side of your head, and when the racket reaches the lowest part of its movement, you will feel the stretch in the back of your arms.

CAUTION

It's a good idea to start from a stable position; keep your back perpendicular to the floor, without overly exaggerating the curve in your lumbar vertebrae while your friend pulls. Your helper will need to remain attentive to your feedback and pull gradually and carefully.

INDICATION

For regular or intense players, especially if they use powerful one-handed backhand shots, since these involve the sudden extension of the elbow and shoulder and the consequent intense involvement of the triceps brachii. This muscle, particularly the long head, can feel the effects and cause discomfort and even become injured in the absence of adequate warm-up and stretching.

Pull with Wrist Extension

START

Stand with one arm forward and extend your elbow so that your hand is in supination, like a bowl, with your fingers pointing straight ahead. Use your other hand to hold the first one, pincer-like, so that your four fingers are together on the palm and your thumb contacts the back of your hand.

TECHNIQUE

Use the holding hand to pull the other one downward, producing wrist extension so that the palm remains facing forward with your fingers pointing downward. The elbow on the side being stretched should remain straight, and you will feel the stretch in the front of your forearm.

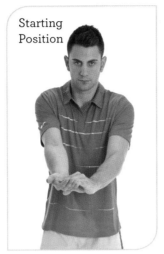

Starting Position

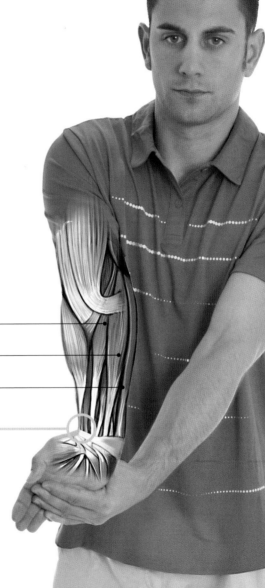

flexor carpi radialis

palmaris longus

flexor carpi ulnaris

Keep your wrist and elbow straight.

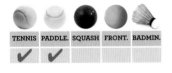

TENNIS	PADDLE.	SQUASH	FRONT.	BADMIN.
✔	✔			

LEVEL	SETS	DURATION
BEGINNER	2	15 s
INTERMEDIATE	2	20 s
ADVANCED	2	20 s

CAUTION

Make sure that your elbow and wrist come into complete extension simultaneously. If you feel joint pain in your wrist or any other discomfort unrelated to muscle tension, reduce the force from the hand doing the pulling.

INDICATION

For players who feel tension in the front of the forearm or the middle of the elbow, or who have previously suffered from golfer's elbow. In contrast to epicondylitis, this tends to affect advanced players who play hard, and it results principally from the repetition of shots such as the tennis serve, the topspin forehand, and others, which are especially hard on the wrist flexor muscles.

Bilateral with Inverted Support

Starting Position

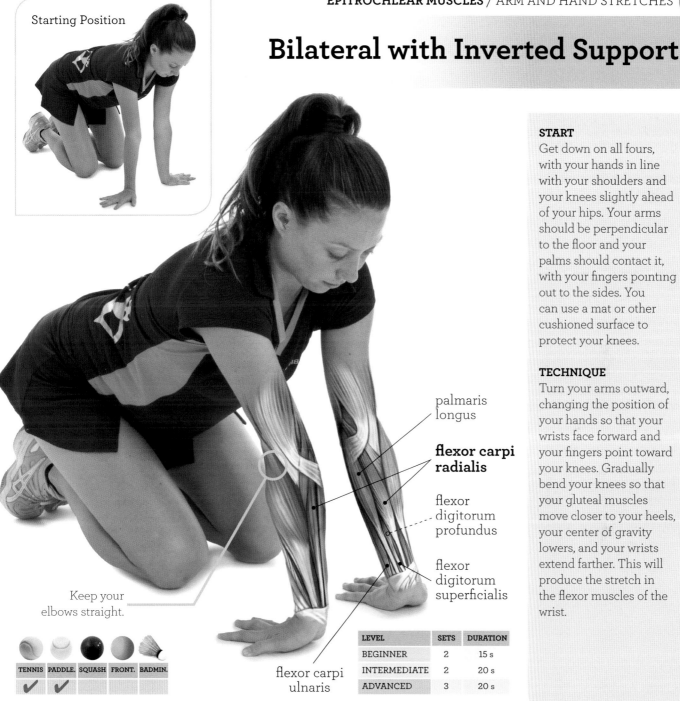

palmaris longus

flexor carpi radialis

flexor digitorum profundus

flexor digitorum superficialis

Keep your elbows straight.

flexor carpi ulnaris

TENNIS	PADDLE.	SQUASH	FRONT.	BADMIN.
✔	✔			

START
Get down on all fours, with your hands in line with your shoulders and your knees slightly ahead of your hips. Your arms should be perpendicular to the floor and your palms should contact it, with your fingers pointing out to the sides. You can use a mat or other cushioned surface to protect your knees.

TECHNIQUE
Turn your arms outward, changing the position of your hands so that your wrists face forward and your fingers point toward your knees. Gradually bend your knees so that your gluteal muscles move closer to your heels, your center of gravity lowers, and your wrists extend farther. This will produce the stretch in the flexor muscles of the wrist.

LEVEL	SETS	DURATION
BEGINNER	2	15 s
INTERMEDIATE	2	20 s
ADVANCED	3	20 s

CAUTION
You must extend your wrists slowly; maintain control as you lower your body and make sure you can stop the movement at any time if any risk manifests itself, such as the appearance of pain in the wrists or reaching their maximum extension.

INDICATION
For players who feel discomfort in the front of their forearm or the middle of their elbow, since these may be a sign of strain in the flexor muscles of the wrist. Also for prevention of epitrocleitis or golfer's elbow in advanced players who play for several hours every day—especially tennis players because of the greater burden on the wrist flexor muscles caused by certain shots, such as the serve and topspin forehand, among others.

Pull with Wrist Bend

START

Stand with both arms held out in front of you. Straighten your elbows, keep your wrists in a neutral position, and move both shoulders forward so that your hands are together. Hold your hands palms down and grasp one hand with the other so that all four fingers are on the back and your thumb is on the palm in a pincer hold.

TECHNIQUE

Pull downward on the hand being stretched so that your wrist is bent and your fingers point downward. Then apply a slight internal rotation so that your fingers point outward. If you keep the elbow on the side being stretched straight, you will feel the tension in the upper part of your forearm, and you may even be able to see the shape of the muscles beneath the skin.

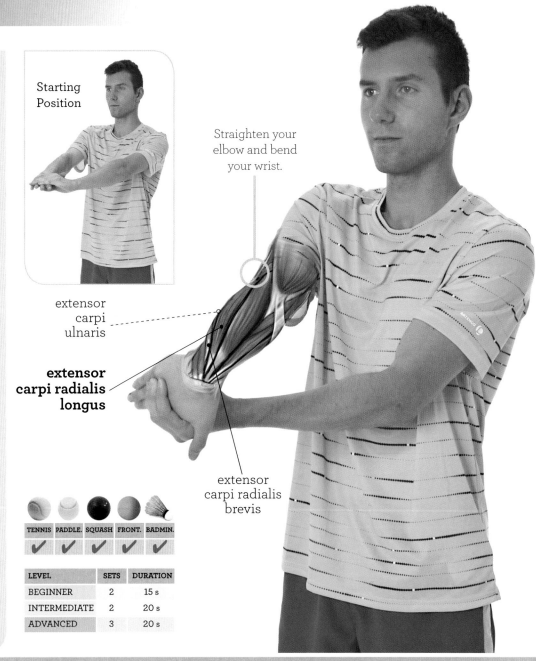

Starting Position

Straighten your elbow and bend your wrist.

extensor carpi ulnaris

extensor carpi radialis longus

extensor carpi radialis brevis

TENNIS	PADDLE.	SQUASH	FRONT.	BADMIN.
✔	✔	✔	✔	✔

LEVEL	SETS	DURATION
BEGINNER	2	15 s
INTERMEDIATE	2	20 s
ADVANCED	3	20 s

CAUTION

Do not use excessive force as you pull on your wrist, and do the movement slowly so you can stop it in time if you feel any discomfort in the joint. Remember that the feeling of muscle tension will not be as noticeable as in other muscle groups or stretches.

INDICATION

For players who experience discomfort in the rear of the forearms or the lateral epicondyle of the elbow, and for people who have previously had epicondylitis or tennis elbow. This pain may appear through repeated use of the backhand, especially if the wrist and elbow are used more than the shoulder. Hitting the ball when it is still in front of the body, along with stretching, may help prevent epicondylitis.

Dorsal Support and Wrist Bend

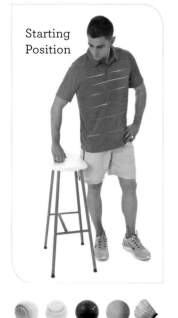

Starting Position

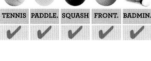

TENNIS	PADDLE.	SQUASH	FRONT.	BADMIN.
✓	✓	✓	✓	✓

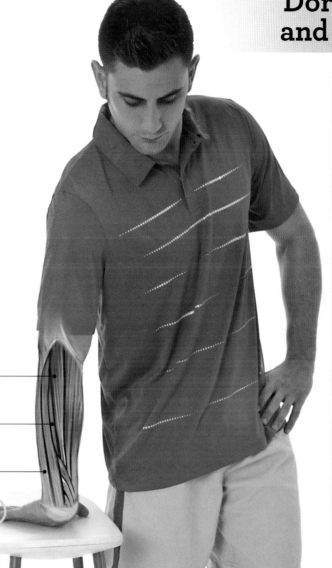

extensor carpi radialis longus

extensor carpi radialis brevis

extensor carpi ulnaris

You fingers face rearward and outward.

START

Use a small, flat, raised surface on which you can place your hand. You can use a stool, a table, or similar item with a height between your knee and your hips. Rest your fingers on the surface without applying any pressure.

TECHNIQUE

Straighten your elbow and bend the wrist of the hand resting on the surface so that the back of your hand contacts the top of the stool and your fingers point rearward. Increase the pronation in your forearm to increase the degree of the stretch by moving the tips of your fingers away from your body.

LEVEL	SETS	DURATION
BEGINNER	2	15 s
INTERMEDIATE	2	20 s
ADVANCED	3	20 s

CAUTION

Remember that the wrist is a joint that has great mobility, plus it is very complex and relatively fragile, so don't apply too much force too abruptly. Be aware of any joint discomfort when you reach the end of the stretch.

INDICATION

For players who have experienced epicondylitis or tennis elbow, or who feel discomfort in the extensor muscles of the wrist; this may arise from the repeated use of the one-hand backhand, especially if it is done very late or the wrist and elbow are used more than the shoulder.

Finger Extension

START
Stand with your elbows bent about 90°, your shoulders in internal rotation, and your hands in front of your upper body with your palms facing you but without contacting your abdomen. Fold your hands and put the tips of your thumbs together.

TECHNIQUE
Place your hands in pronation so that your palms face forward and down at the same time you straighten your elbows. You should keep your hands folded to achieve the maximum stretch in the flexor muscles of the wrist and fingers. You will feel the stretch in the palms of your hands and the front part of your fingers, especially at the base.

	TENNIS	PADDLE.	SQUASH	FRONT.	BADMIN.
	✔	✔	✔	✔	✔

LEVEL	SETS	DURATION
BEGINNER	2	15 s
INTERMEDIATE	2	20 s
ADVANCED	3	20 s

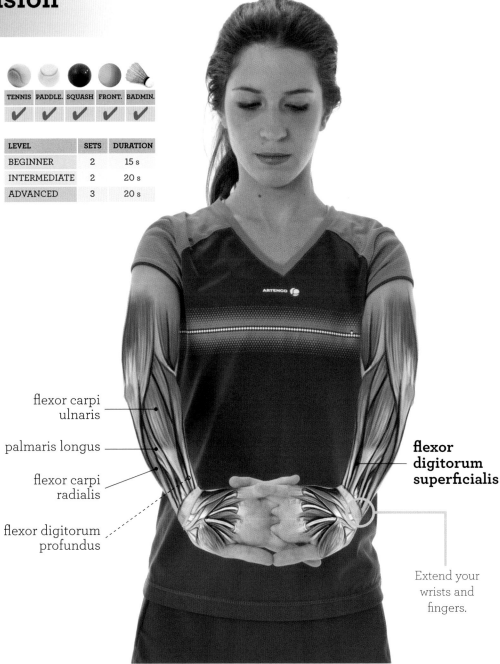

flexor carpi ulnaris

palmaris longus

flexor carpi radialis

flexor digitorum profundus

flexor digitorum superficialis

Extend your wrists and fingers.

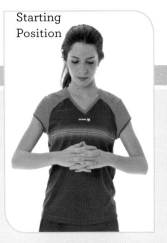

Starting Position

CAUTION
Be careful with the force you apply to your fingers, since their joints are small and relatively fragile. Remember that the stretch may produce discomfort, but not pain.

INDICATION
For all players of racket and paddle sports because of the constant work performed by the flexor muscles of the wrist and fingers in the grip, which involves prolonged effort and few pauses or rests; especially for athletes who train or compete for several hours a day.

Inverted Prayer Position

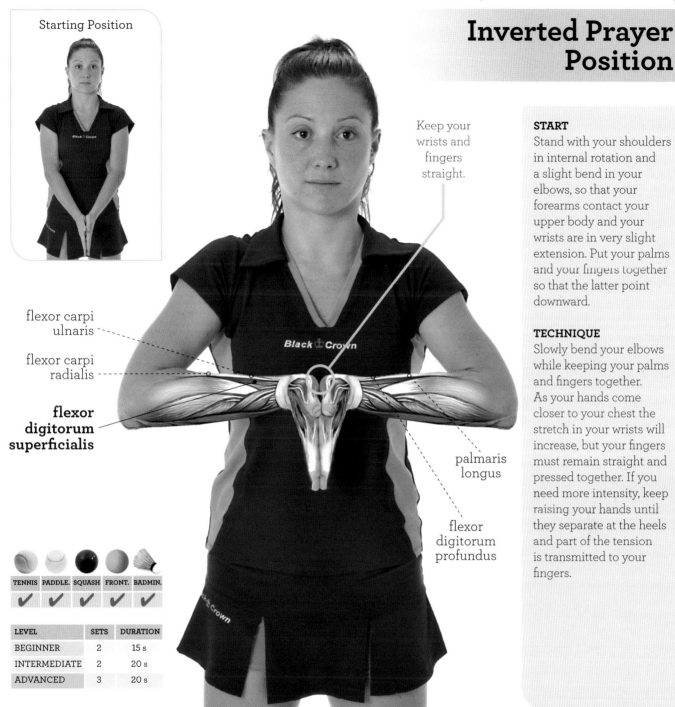

Starting Position

Keep your wrists and fingers straight.

flexor carpi ulnaris

flexor carpi radialis

flexor digitorum superficialis

palmaris longus

flexor digitorum profundus

START
Stand with your shoulders in internal rotation and a slight bend in your elbows, so that your forearms contact your upper body and your wrists are in very slight extension. Put your palms and your fingers together so that the latter point downward.

TECHNIQUE
Slowly bend your elbows while keeping your palms and fingers together. As your hands come closer to your chest the stretch in your wrists will increase, but your fingers must remain straight and pressed together. If you need more intensity, keep raising your hands until they separate at the heels and part of the tension is transmitted to your fingers.

TENNIS	PADDLE.	SQUASH	FRONT.	BADMIN.
✔	✔	✔	✔	✔

LEVEL	SETS	DURATION
BEGINNER	2	15 s
INTERMEDIATE	2	20 s
ADVANCED	3	20 s

CAUTION
Apply moderate force when stretching your wrists and fingers. Keep in mind that you should never cross the line between discomfort and pain; that way you will preserve the health of your muscles and joints.

INDICATION
For all players of racket and paddle sports because of the almost continual gripping force used in training and competition, especially over long periods of time, as well as for athletes who practice hard or play or train for several hours a day.

Thumb Pull

START

Place one hand in front of your body, with the palm facing inside and your fingers straight, together, and pointing forward. Your thumb should point upward. Using your free hand, grasp your raised thumb so that your fingers wrap around it and you hold it in your closed fist.

TECHNIQUE

Carefully pull your thumb rearward, keeping your hand and forearm in their original position so that the only movement is in the hand being stretched, in extending the thumb and its carpometacarpal, metacarpophalangeal, and interphalangeal joints. You will feel the tension at the base of your thumb and the space between your thumb and index finger.

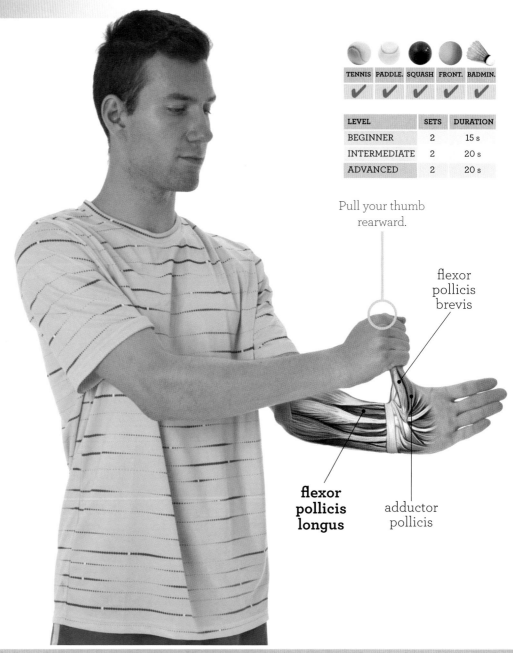

		TENNIS	PADDLE.	SQUASH	FRONT.	BADMIN.
		✔	✔	✔	✔	✔

LEVEL	SETS	DURATION
BEGINNER	2	15 s
INTERMEDIATE	2	20 s
ADVANCED	2	20 s

Pull your thumb rearward.

flexor pollicis brevis

flexor pollicis longus

adductor pollicis

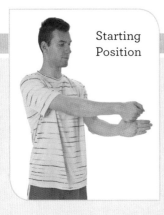

Starting Position

CAUTION

Remember that the force applied to the thumb or any other digit should be limited and applied gradually, to avoid injuring your joints.

INDICATION

For all players of racket and paddle sports, to keep the flexor and adductor muscles of the thumb in good condition, given the sustained work that they perform in the grip during play and training; especially for intense players or ones who have suffered from De Quervain's tenosynovitis.

Inverted Rhombus Position

Starting Position

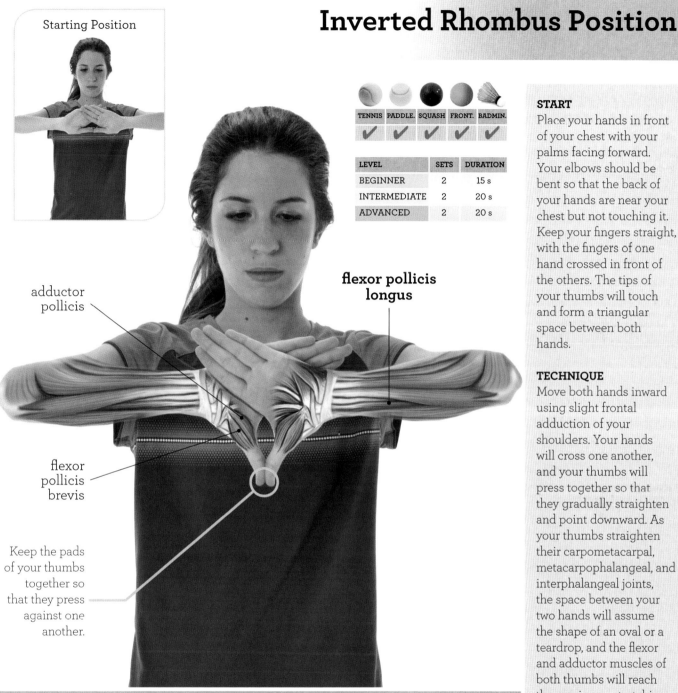

TENNIS	PADDLE.	SQUASH	FRONT.	BADMIN.
✓	✓	✓	✓	✓

LEVEL	SETS	DURATION
BEGINNER	2	15 s
INTERMEDIATE	2	20 s
ADVANCED	2	20 s

adductor pollicis

flexor pollicis longus

flexor pollicis brevis

Keep the pads of your thumbs together so that they press against one another.

START
Place your hands in front of your chest with your palms facing forward. Your elbows should be bent so that the back of your hands are near your chest but not touching it. Keep your fingers straight, with the fingers of one hand crossed in front of the others. The tips of your thumbs will touch and form a triangular space between both hands.

TECHNIQUE
Move both hands inward using slight frontal adduction of your shoulders. Your hands will cross one another, and your thumbs will press together so that they gradually straighten and point downward. As your thumbs straighten their carpometacarpal, metacarpophalangeal, and interphalangeal joints, the space between your two hands will assume the shape of an oval or a teardrop, and the flexor and adductor muscles of both thumbs will reach the maximum stretching point.

CAUTION
Remember that the fingers and their joints are relatively fragile, and it is quite easy to cross the pain threshold, which is the prelude to injury; you need to be careful and increase the pressure slowly.

INDICATION
For players of racket and paddle sports, to offset the constant work performed by the flexors and adductors of the thumb while holding the grip, and especially for players whose practice is intense or who have suffered from De Quervain's tenosynovitis.

Punch Position

START
Reach forward with one arm, with your elbow almost completely straight and your thumb inside your clenched fist; this will put you into a position similar to the end of a straight punch. Grasp your first hand with the free one so that your fingers rest on the back of your hand and knuckles. Your thumb should press on the middle phalanges of your fingers in a pincer hold.

TECHNIQUE
Using your gripping hand, pull the other one downward and rearward while keeping your fist clenched. This will produce flexion in your wrist; along with the flexion in all of your finger joints, this will accomplish the stretch in your wrist extensor muscles and your fingers. You will feel the tension in the back of your wrist and hand.

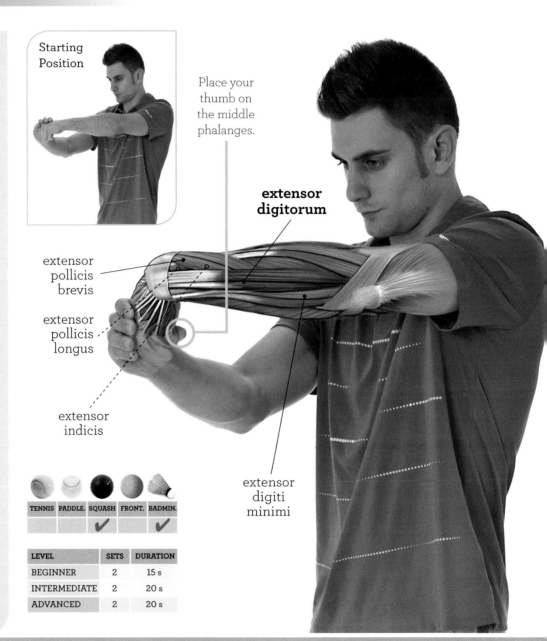

Starting Position

Place your thumb on the middle phalanges.

extensor digitorum

extensor pollicis brevis

extensor pollicis longus

extensor indicis

extensor digiti minimi

	TENNIS	PADDLE.	SQUASH	FRONT.	BADMIN.
			✔		✔

LEVEL	SETS	DURATION
BEGINNER	2	15 s
INTERMEDIATE	2	20 s
ADVANCED	2	20 s

CAUTION
Use care in applying tension to your wrists, since they are complex joints and it is relatively easy to injure them by applying excessive or sudden force. It is preferable to increase the duration rather than the intensity of an exercise.

INDICATION
For athletes who use rackets or paddles, especially those whose technical moves involve the wrist more, such as a one-hand backhand. This particular use of wrist movement commonly occurs in badminton and squash players, as well as others.

Wrist and Finger Bend

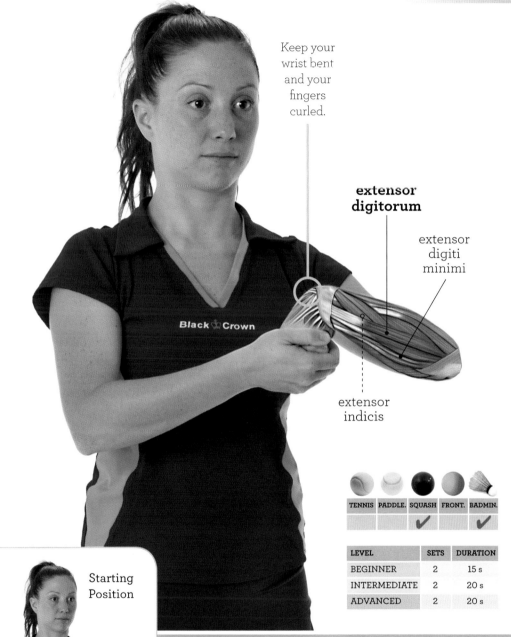

Keep your wrist bent and your fingers curled.

extensor digitorum

extensor digiti minimi

extensor indicis

Starting Position

START

Bend your shoulders slightly and rotate them to the inside. Bend your elbows to about 90° so that both hands are in front of your chest with your thumbs near it. Make a fist with the hand being stretched while your keep your wrist in a neutral position. Use your free hand to cover the fingers, knuckles, and back of your other hand.

TECHNIQUE

Pull the held hand downward, producing flexion in the wrist; keep your fingers bent and your hand in a fist. Your forearm should remain in the original position or rise slightly as your wrist bends. At the end of the motion, you will feel the tension from the stretch in the back of your wrist and hand.

TENNIS	PADDLE.	SQUASH	FRONT.	BADMIN.
		✔		✔

LEVEL	SETS	DURATION
BEGINNER	2	15 s
INTERMEDIATE	2	20 s
ADVANCED	2	20 s

CAUTION

If you do not feel tension when you reach the end of the movement, do not increase the pressure on your wrist, since that could injure it and you would get nothing for any increase in the intensity of the stretch.

INDICATION

For athletes who use rackets or paddles in their disciplines, especially for those who use lots of wrist extension in the one-handed backhand, as in squash or badminton, especially if the play is intense.

HIP STRETCHES

Like any physical activity that involves running or using the legs to change position, racket and paddle sports place huge demands on the muscles that move the hip joint. Even though it appears that these disciplines don't involve overly lengthy moves, or that the total distance covered by the end of a match doesn't amount to much, the work certainly is intense because of the speed, the force, and the variety of the moves. Racket and paddle sports involve not only running forward, but also to the sides, long single strides to reach the ball and return to the starting position, plus jumps. Individual strides, jumps, running, and the tennis serve and overhead place heavy demands on the hip extensor and flexor muscles, including the gluteus maximus and the iliopsoas (the psoas major and iliac) because of their almost instantaneous series of extensions and contractions. In addition, lateral runs and the slides that occur on certain surfaces involve intense work from the abductor and adductor muscles of the hips, such as the gluteus medius and minimus, the tensor fasciae latae, and the long, short, and great adductors. So in order to prevent strain, injury, pain, and numbness and to improve performance and recovery, both stretches and strength work are essential.

ADDUCTOR MAGNUS

This muscle originates at the lower branch of the os pubis, the sciatic branch, and the sciatic tuberosity, and it inserts at the linea aspera femoris (rough line of the femur), at the proximal two thirds of the diaphysis. Its main function is adduction of the hip joint, but it also participates to a lesser degree in hip extension, flexion, and rotation.

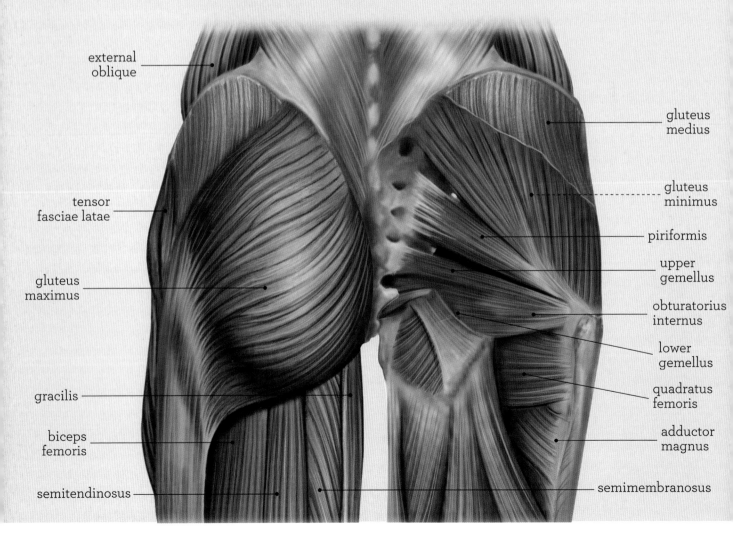

external oblique

gluteus medius

tensor fasciae latae

gluteus minimus

piriformis

gluteus maximus

upper gemellus

obturatorius internus

lower gemellus

gracilis

quadratus femoris

biceps femoris

adductor magnus

semitendinosus

semimembranosus

ADDUCTOR LONGUS

This muscle originates at the upper branch of the os pubis, and it inserts at the linea aspera femoris, at the middle third of the diaphysis. Its main function is hip adduction, although it participates to a lesser degree in its flexion and rotation.

ADDUCTOR BREVIS

This muscle originates at the lower branch of the os pubis, and it inserts at the linea aspera femoris, at the proximal third of the diaphysis. Its function is hip adduction, and to a lesser degree, hip flexion and rotation.

GLUTEUS MAXIMUS

This muscle originates at the rear face of the sacral bone, the rear face of the os ilii, the thoracolumbar fascia, and the sacrotuberal ligament, and it inserts at the iliotibial tract and the gluteal tuberosity of the femur. Its main functions are extension and abduction of the hip, although it also participates in its external rotation and adduction.

GLUTEUS MEDIUS

This muscle originates at the rear face of the os ilii, and it inserts at the trochanter major femoris. Its main function is hip abduction, but it participates in its flexion, extension, and rotation, both external and internal.

GLUTEUS MINIMUS

This muscle originates at the rear face of the os ilii, below the gluteus maximus and gluteus medius. Its insertion is at the major trochanter of the femur, and it shares functions with the gluteus medius.

ILIACUS

This muscle originates at the iliac fossa, and it inserts at the lesser trochanter of the femur. Its main functions are hip flexion and external rotation.

PSOAS MAJOR

This muscle originates at the bodies and intervertebral discs of vertebrae T12 to L4, as well as at the transverse apophyses of vertebrae L1 to L5. Its insertion is at the lesser trochanter of the femur, and it shares functions with the iliac muscle.

TENSOR FASCIAE LATAE

This muscle originates at the upper anterior iliac spine, and it inserts at the iliotibial tract. Its main functions are hip abduction, flexion, and internal rotation.

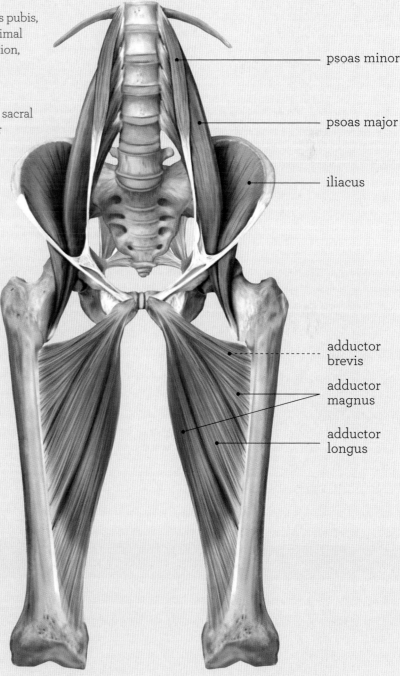

psoas minor

psoas major

iliacus

adductor brevis

adductor magnus

adductor longus

Knight's Position

START

Take a position resting on one knee and one foot. You will need to rest the sole of one foot on the floor so that your knee and hip are bent to 90°. The trailing leg should start from a position in which the thigh is in line with your upper body and your knee is bent about 90° and in contact with the floor. Your foot will be behind you and resting on your toes or your instep.

TECHNIQUE

Move your upper body ahead without moving your original support points, so that your forward knee bends further and the rear one straightens. As your center of gravity moves forward and downward, the hip of the support leg will keep straightening, producing the stretch in the flexor muscles and a sensation of muscle tension in the groin on the side being stretched.

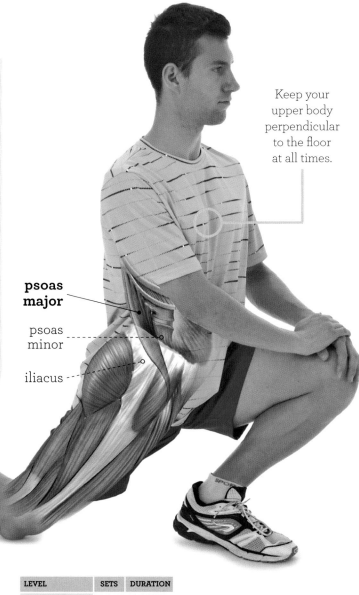

Keep your upper body perpendicular to the floor at all times.

psoas major

psoas minor

iliacus

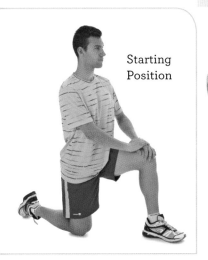

Starting Position

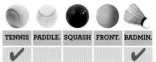

TENNIS	PADDLE.	SQUASH	FRONT.	BADMIN.
✔				✔

LEVEL	SETS	DURATION
BEGINNER	2	20 s
INTERMEDIATE	2	25 s
ADVANCED	3	25 s

CAUTION

It's a good idea to use a mat or a cushioned surface under the support knee, especially if you are doing the stretch on a rough or uneven surface. That way you will avoid discomfort in the joint and any skin injuries due to pressure.

INDICATION

Particularly for players who make high shots involving jumps, as with the serve in tennis and some overhead shots, because of the sudden extension and contraction that some muscles of the anterior chain undergo, including the flexors of the hip.

Hip Extension with Fitness Ball

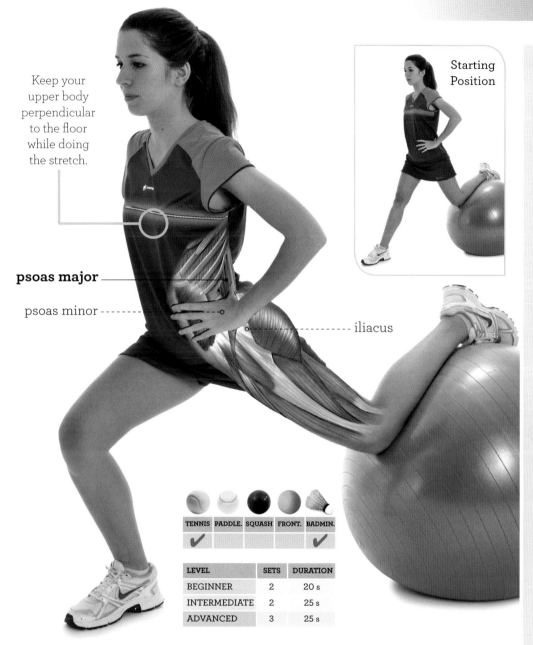

Keep your upper body perpendicular to the floor while doing the stretch.

psoas major

psoas minor

iliacus

Starting Position

TENNIS	PADDLE.	SQUASH	FRONT.	BADMIN.
✔				✔

LEVEL	SETS	DURATION
BEGINNER	2	20 s
INTERMEDIATE	2	25 s
ADVANCED	3	25 s

START

For this stretch you will need a fitness ball or some other item of similar height that can serve the same support function. Place the fitness ball behind you and rest one leg on it so that your shin and instep contact it; your other foot will contact the floor slightly ahead of your upper body. You can place your hands on your hips or use your arms to improve your stability and keep your balance.

TECHNIQUE

Bend the forward knee to about 90°. This will move your center of gravity forward and downward, producing extension in the hip being stretched. Keep your rear support leg in place, and the fitness ball will move slightly as you do the exercise. You will feel the stretch in you hip flexor muscles and groin.

CAUTION

The fitness ball is a very versatile item in doing other exercises besides stretching, but its spherical shape lacks stability, so you should take some time to get used to it if you decide to use it, and make sure you are in a solid position before starting the movement.

INDICATION

For players of racket and paddle sports who regularly make high shots involving a jump, such as the tennis serve and overheads, among others, because of the extension and contraction that the anterior muscle chain experiences.

Low Stride

START

Stand with one foot ahead of the other. Both knees should be slightly bent, with your upper body leaning forward. You can rest both hands on your forward knee for added stability and reduced effort while doing the exercise.

TECHNIQUE

Slide your trailing foot farther to the rear while straightening the corresponding knee. This will lower your center of gravity, extend your hip, and stretch your flexor muscles. If you want to increase the intensity of the stretch, keep straightening your elbows and position your upper body more perpendicular to the floor until the muscle tension is appropriate for your level of flexibility.

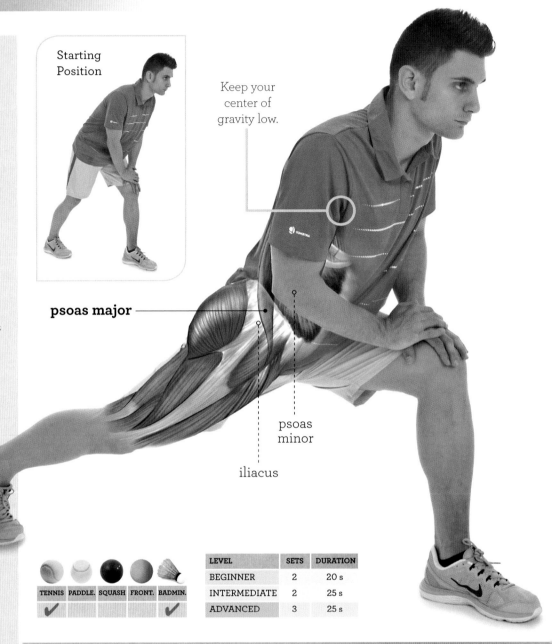

Starting Position

Keep your center of gravity low.

psoas major

psoas minor

iliacus

TENNIS	PADDLE.	SQUASH	FRONT.	BADMIN.
✓				✓

LEVEL	SETS	DURATION
BEGINNER	2	20 s
INTERMEDIATE	2	25 s
ADVANCED	3	25 s

CAUTION

Start from a stable position, with your hands planted solidly on your knee. Remember that the first phase of the technique is enough for many people, and if you need to, you should increase only the intensity of the stretch, but without exceeding the limits. It takes time to improve flexibility.

INDICATION

For players who use high shots involving a jump, such as the serve in tennis, and overheads, which are more common in tennis and badminton, because of the involvement of the hip flexor muscles and others.

Crossed Leg Pull

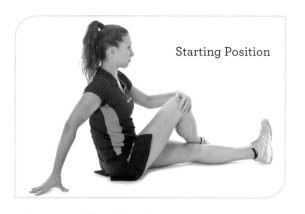

Starting Position

TENNIS	PADDLE.	SQUASH	FRONT.	BADMIN.
✔	✔	✔	✔	✔

LEVEL	SETS	DURATION
BEGINNER	2	25 s
INTERMEDIATE	3	25 s
ADVANCED	3	30 s

START

Sit down with one leg straight so that it rests on the back of your thigh, calf, and heel. Bend the other knee to an angle less than 90° and cross that leg over the other one so that the sole of your foot contacts the floor. The hand on the side of the straight leg should contact the bent knee, and the other hand will contact the floor behind your upper body to stabilize your position.

TECHNIQUE

While keeping your foot in the same support position, use your hand to pull your bent knee toward the inside, which will produce greater adduction in your hip. As the movement progresses, you will feel the muscle tension from the stretch in the side of the gluteal muscle of the crossed leg.

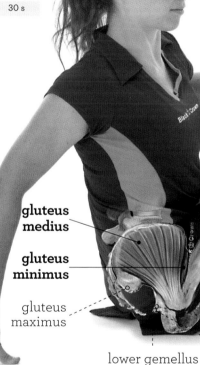

Pull on your knee in order to cross the thigh being stretched over the other one.

gluteus medius

gluteus minimus

gluteus maximus

upper gemellus

lower gemellus

piriformis

CAUTION

This exercise does not involve any difficulty or specific risk, since it uses a simple technique on a large, sturdy joint. All you have to do is start from a stable position, with a solid hold and support points, and avoid going beyond the discomfort involved in any stretch.

INDICATION

For players of racket and paddle sports because of the constant use of movement to the sides, jumps, and quick starts to reach the ball or shuttlecock, which involve the hip abductor and extensor muscles. Especially for players who are susceptible to muscle discomfort or strain in the gluteal muscles.

Supine Knee Pull

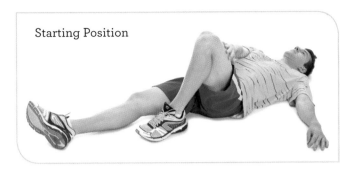

Starting Position

START

Lie down on your back with your head resting on the floor. Keep one leg straight and relaxed, and bend the knee of the other leg so that the sole of your foot contacts the floor. The arm on the side of the raised leg should be straight out to the side at about a 45° angle to your upper body to help maintain a stable position while doing the exercise. Your other hand should rest on the raised thigh and near your knee.

TECHNIQUE

Slide the hand on your thigh upward as far as your knee; then grasp it firmly and pull it toward the inside; this will produce adduction of the hip and will slightly increase its bend. With the additional hip abduction, the stretch will make itself felt in the side and the back of the gluteus.

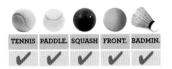

					LEVEL	SETS	DURATION
TENNIS	PADDLE.	SQUASH	FRONT.	BADMIN.	BEGINNER	2	25 s
✔	✔	✔	✔	✔	INTERMEDIATE	3	25 s
					ADVANCED	3	30 s

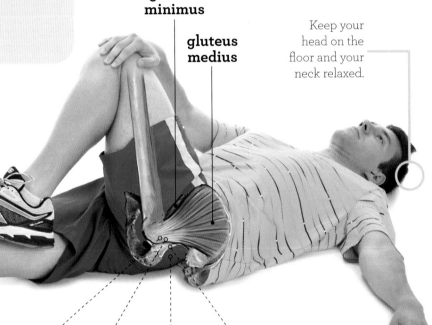

gluteus minimus

gluteus medius

Keep your head on the floor and your neck relaxed.

lower gemellus   upper gemellus   gluteus maximus   piriformis

CAUTION

Even though in many exercises it's a good idea to look at the area being moved to make sure that the exercise is being done correctly, in this case keep your head on the floor to avoid tension.

INDICATION

For athletes who play racket or paddle sports, to avoid strain or muscle discomfort in the gluteal muscles; this can occur, for example, from the repeated use of jumps, movements to the side, and sudden starts, especially in athletes who play hard or who play or train for several hours a day.

Supine Pull to Chest

Starting Position

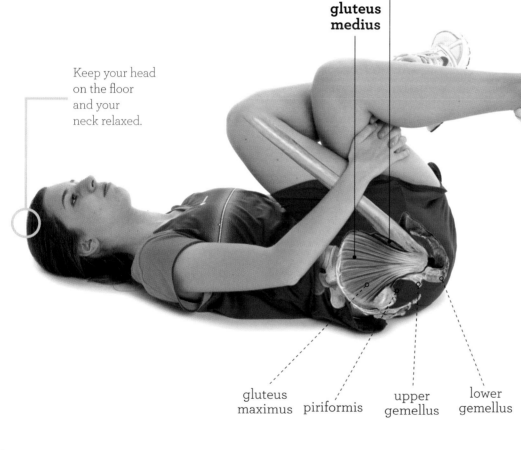

LEVEL	SETS	DURATION
BEGINNER	2	25 s
INTERMEDIATE	3	25 s
ADVANCED	3	30 s

TENNIS ✔ PADDLE. ✔ SQUASH FRONT. ✔ BADMIN.

gluteus minimus

gluteus medius

Keep your head on the floor and your neck relaxed.

gluteus maximus   piriformis   upper gemellus   lower gemellus

START

Lie down on your back and rest your head on the floor. Bend the hip and knee of one leg so that the sole of your foot rests on the floor. Cross the leg being stretched over the other one and bend your knee so that it contacts and rests on the opposite thigh. Place both hands on the thigh of the leg that contacts the floor.

TECHNIQUE

Bend your hips, raising your foot from the floor. Move your arms forward and fold your hands beneath the forward thigh. Without changing your grip or the crossed-legs position, pull with both hands by bending your elbows, drawing your thighs toward your chest. You will feel the stretch in the gluteal muscle of the leg that is closer to your chest.

CAUTION

Remember to keep your head on the floor as long as possible during the stretch so you avoid creating tension in the anterior muscles of your neck and cervical vertebrae.

INDICATION

For athletes in racket and paddle sports, in order to prevent discomfort or muscle strain in the gluteal muscles, which may result from the quick starts, jumps, and strides with a return to the starting position that are necessary during play to reach a ball or a shuttlecock.

Supine Unilateral Pull to Chest

START

Lie down on your back with both legs straight. Bend one hip and knee on the same side so that your thigh is perpendicular to the floor. Reach forward with your arms and place your hands on your leg so that your palms are to the sides and your fingers reach around to the front to provide a good hold.

TECHNIQUE

Pull your leg toward your chest by bending your elbows, producing the maximum bend in the leg being stretched. As your thigh comes closer to your chest the stretch will be felt increasingly in your gluteal muscle. When this feels adequate, hold the position for the duration appropriate to your level and your goals.

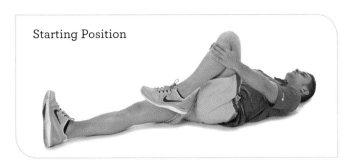

Starting Position

Keep your head on the floor and your neck relaxed.

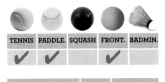

TENNIS	PADDLE.	SQUASH	FRONT.	BADMIN.
✔	✔		✔	

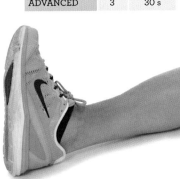

LEVEL	SETS	DURATION
BEGINNER	2	25 s
INTERMEDIATE	3	25 s
ADVANCED	3	30 s

gluteus maximus   gluteus medius   gluteus minimus

CAUTION

Sometimes it is appropriate to watch an exercise to make sure it is done correctly; however, in this case, keep your neck relaxed and your head on the floor for the duration of the stretch. This will prevent tension in the area of your cervical vertebrae.

INDICATION

For players who experience or who have experienced tension or muscle strain in the gluteal muscles, as well as for those who wish to prevent such problems, especially if fast starts and short runs are common in their discipline.

Supine Butterfly

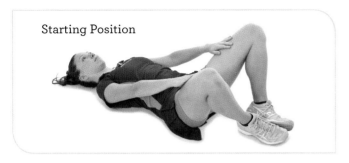

Starting Position

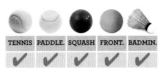

	TENNIS	PADDLE.	SQUASH	FRONT.	BADMIN.
	✔	✔	✔	✔	✔

LEVEL	SETS	DURATION
BEGINNER	2	20 s
INTERMEDIATE	3	20 s
ADVANCED	3	25 s

START
Lie down on your back with your head resting on the floor and your neck relaxed. Bend your knees and keep your feet together and contacting the floor. At this point use hip abduction to move your knees apart so that the soles of both feet face each other. Reach out with your arms and place your hands on the inside of your thighs.

TECHNIQUE
Push your thighs downward with your hands so that your knees separate and gradually approach the floor. This forced hip abduction will stretch your adductor muscles, and you will feel the tension along the inside of your thighs, and especially in the strip near your groin.

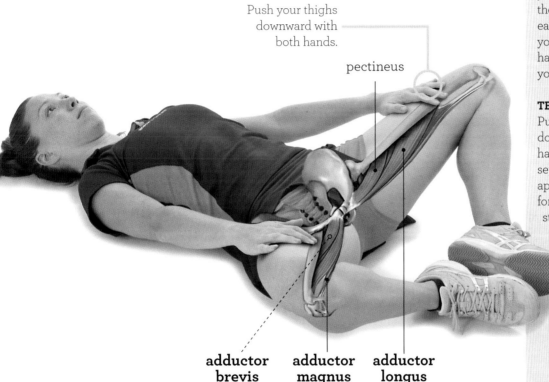

Push your thighs downward with both hands.

pectineus

adductor brevis

adductor magnus

adductor longus

CAUTION
This position may cause joint discomfort in your groin if you use too much pressure. So use moderate, gradual force. Also remember that it's a good idea to keep your head resting on the floor.

INDICATION
For players of paddle and racket sports because of the repeated use of lateral moves and long strides that put the hip adductor muscles under considerable muscle tension as a result of stretching and contracting. Especially recommended for players who are susceptible to injuries of the hip adductor muscles.

Hip Abduction with Fitness Ball

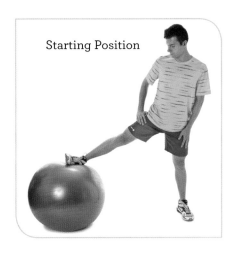

Starting Position

START

Use a fitness ball or some other item of similar height to do this exercise, and take a position next to it. Raise one leg to the side through hip abduction; rest the inside of your foot on the top of the fitness ball. Make sure that your position is solid, and place your hands on your thighs to help maintain the final position.

TECHNIQUE

Bend the knee and the hip of the leg in contact with the floor, lowering your center of gravity and accentuating the hip abduction in the other leg; keep the inside of your foot on top of the fitness ball. You will feel the stretch on the inside of the raised thigh, and more particularly in the area near your groin.

pectineus

gracilis

adductor major **adductor longus** **adductor brevis**

Place your hands on your thighs for support.

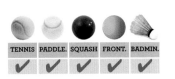

TENNIS	PADDLE.	SQUASH	FRONT.	BADMIN.
✔	✔	✔	✔	✔

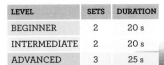

LEVEL	SETS	DURATION
BEGINNER	2	20 s
INTERMEDIATE	2	20 s
ADVANCED	3	25 s

CAUTION

The fitness ball is a versatile item, but you have to get used to using it because its spherical shape makes it unstable and you need to have good balance. Start from a solid, well-balanced position before beginning the movement, and use a separate support if you don't feel secure.

INDICATION

For players of racket and paddle sports because of the common use of lateral movements and fast starts, and the involvement of the hip adductor muscles and others, and especially for players who are prone to experiencing discomfort in the adductors or who play hard.

Static Butterfly

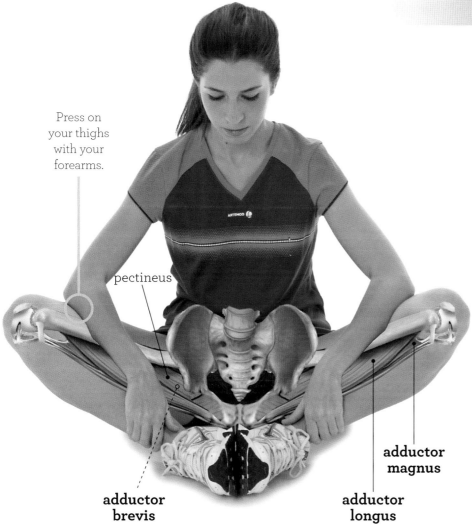

Press on your thighs with your forearms.

pectineus

adductor brevis

adductor magnus

adductor longus

START
Sit down on the floor with your knees and hips bent, keeping the soles of your feet in contact with one another. Slide your forearms over the inside of your thighs and calves until your hands reach your ankles, and keep them in this position. Hold your legs just above your ankles so that the palms of both hands face outward.

TECHNIQUE
Push downward on your thighs with your forearms; this will produce abduction in both hips. Keep the soles of your feet in contact with one another. You can bend your upper body slightly and use the weight to help you. You will feel the tension from the stretch from your groin to the inside of your knees, and it will gradually decrease with distance from your groin.

Starting Position

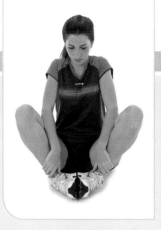

	TENNIS	PADDLE.	SQUASH	FRONT.	BADMIN.
	✓	✓	✓	✓	✓

LEVEL	SETS	DURATION
BEGINNER	2	20 s
INTERMEDIATE	2	20 s
ADVANCED	3	25 s

CAUTION

Don't apply too much pressure too quickly or suddenly, especially if you are prone to feeling discomfort in your adductors, because of the risk this might entail for the hip adductor muscles.

INDICATION

For athletes in paddle or racket sports because of the repeated use of lateral moves and long strides to reach the ball or shuttlecock, and because of the demands that these moves place on the hip adductor muscles. Especially for athletes who have previously experienced discomfort in these muscles, and for players who train or play hard.

Rear Foot Cross with Helper

START

In order to do this exercise you will need a friend to help you hold the position. You can also use a vertical support. Stand next to your helper and hold his shoulder as you gently move the foot that is closer to him to the rear. Your helper can also hold your arm or shoulder to help you keep your balance.

TECHNIQUE

Shift your rear foot onto its side so that the leg being stretched crosses behind your support leg; the latter should bend at the knee to lower your center of gravity. The rear leg should remain straight to achieve the greatest possible hip adduction and take better advantage of the exercise.

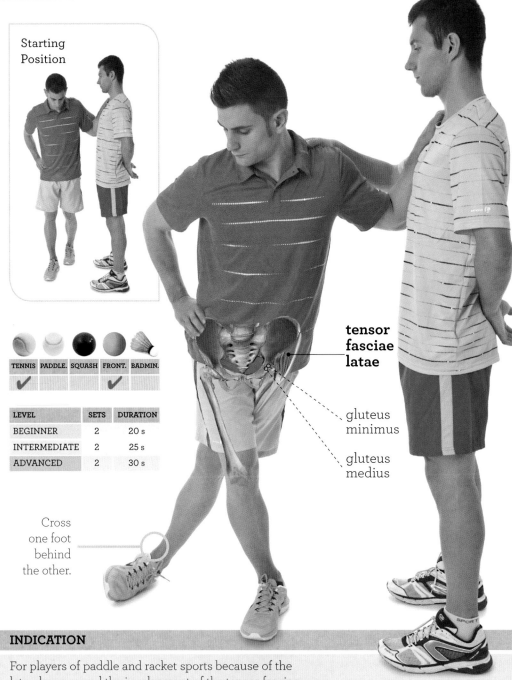

Starting Position

TENNIS	PADDLE.	SQUASH	FRONT.	BADMIN.
✔			✔	

LEVEL	SETS	DURATION
BEGINNER	2	20 s
INTERMEDIATE	2	25 s
ADVANCED	2	30 s

Cross one foot behind the other.

tensor fasciae latae

gluteus minimus

gluteus medius

CAUTION

Make sure that the supports on your leg and your friend are solid and that you have a good hold so you can keep your balance as you perform the exercise and lower your center of gravity.

INDICATION

For players of paddle and racket sports because of the lateral moves and the involvement of the tensor fasciae latae, particularly in recovering the position of the first leg in the direction of the move. Especially for players who have experienced discomfort in the outside of the knee, who have previously had trocanteric bursitis or iliotibial tract syndrome, or who play for long times with fairly long lateral movements.

Supine Rear Hip Adduction

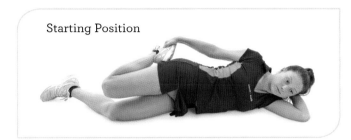

Starting Position

LEVEL	SETS	DURATION
BEGINNER	2	20 s
INTERMEDIATE	2	25 s
ADVANCED	2	30 s

TENNIS PADDLE. SQUASH FRONT. BADMIN.

START

Lie down on your side. Bend your upper knee, trying to bring your heel to your gluteal muscle. Hold your instep with your hand without pulling. Your lower leg should remain relaxed; you can rest your head on your free forearm to reduce the tension in your neck while doing this exercise.

TECHNIQUE

Pull rearward on your instep; this will produce a certain amount of hip extension. Bend your lower hip and knee, and place your free foot onto the opposite knee. Push it downward, trying to move it to the floor and produce hip adduction and the resulting stretch in the tensor fasciae latae, which you will feel slightly.

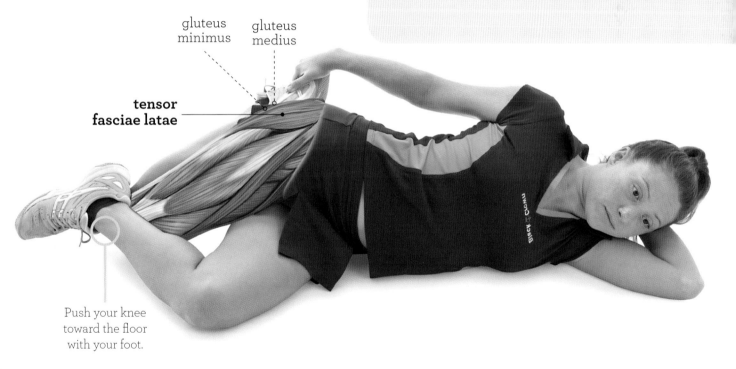

gluteus minimus

gluteus medius

tensor fasciae latae

Push your knee toward the floor with your foot.

CAUTION

For greater effectiveness, make sure to combine the extension and adduction of your hip, omitting none of these actions. Also support your head to achieve a more comfortable and secure position for your head.

INDICATION

For all players of racket and paddle sports because of the repeated use of lateral moves and the demands to which the hip abductor muscles are subjected, as well as for players who have experienced discomfort in the outside of the hip and knee, trocanteric bursitis, or iliotibial tract syndrome.

Knight's Position with Hip Adduction

START

Take a position next to a vertical support and place your hand on it. The height of the support does not matter; it merely must stay in place if subjected to lateral pressure. The thigh closer to the support should be perpendicular to the floor, with your knee bent to 90° and resting on the floor. Your hip and knee farther from the support should be bent to 90° so that your foot rests on the floor.

TECHNIQUE

Move your support foot closer to the support, and then move your whole body toward it while keeping the knee support in place. The knee of that support leg will gradually increase its position of adduction; this will also lower your center of gravity and stretch the tensor fasciae latae.

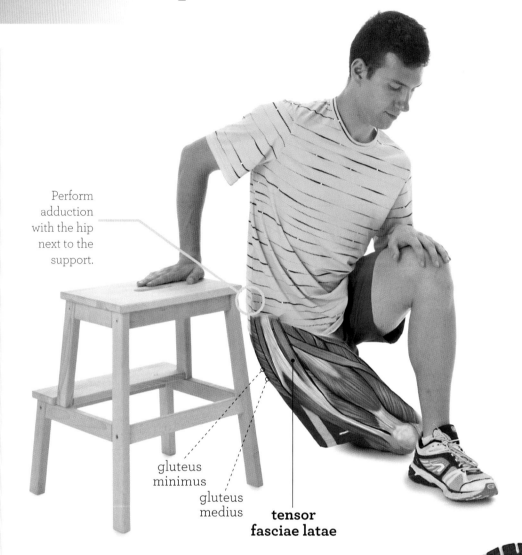

Perform adduction with the hip next to the support.

gluteus minimus

gluteus medius

tensor fasciae latae

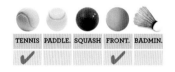

TENNIS	PADDLE.	SQUASH	FRONT.	BADMIN.
✔			✔	

LEVEL	SETS	DURATION
BEGINNER	2	20 s
INTERMEDIATE	2	25 s
ADVANCED	2	30 s

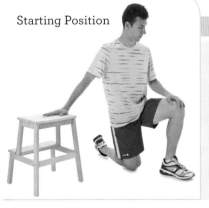

Starting Position

CAUTION

Make sure that you use a solid support, and use a mat, a towel, or some other cushion for your support knee if you feel any discomfort or if you have to do the stretch on a rough surface.

INDICATION

For athletes who play racket or paddle sports because of the importance of the hip abductor muscles due to the repeated use of lateral moves, and for players who feel discomfort in the outside of the knee or hip, or if they have previously felt discomfort related to friction in the iliotibial tract.

Supine Cross

Starting
Position

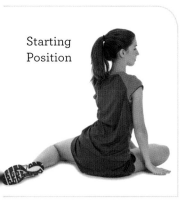

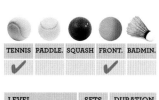

TENNIS	PADDLE.	SQUASH	FRONT.	BADMIN.
✔			✔	

LEVEL	SETS	DURATION
BEGINNER	2	15 s
INTERMEDIATE	2	20 s
ADVANCED	2	25 s

START

Sit down with your back perpendicular to the floor. Move one leg forward, with your hip rotated to the outside and your knee bent so that the outside of your thigh and calf contact the floor. The opposite hip should be in abduction, with your knee bent to 90° so that the inside of your thigh and calf contact the floor.

TECHNIQUE

Bend your upper body forward so that you are lying on your forward thigh. Your hands should slide along the floor in the same direction so that they end up beyond your head. The increased outer rotation and bend in the hip will stretch the piriformis, and you will feel it below your gluteus maximus.

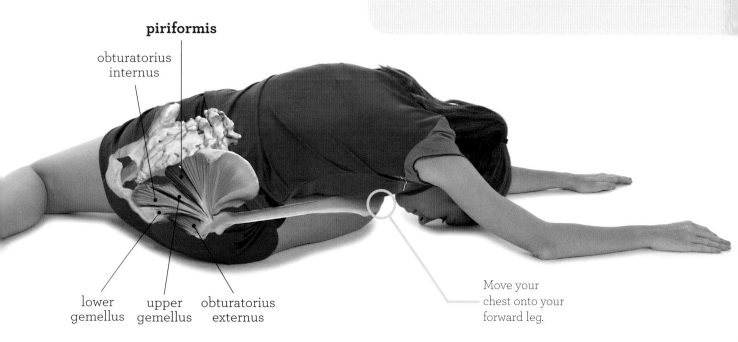

piriformis

obturatorius
internus

lower
gemellus

upper
gemellus

obturatorius
externus

Move your
chest onto your
forward leg.

CAUTION

Do the movement slowly, controlling the downward movement of your upper body; that way you can stop if you experience any discomfort not connected to the muscle tension that accompanies the stretch.

INDICATION

For players who may experience discomfort, pain, or numbness in the back of the thigh, the gluteal muscles, or the lumbar area, which could be due to piriformis syndrome; this is fairly common in runners and athletes who run a lot, such as tennis players and frontenis players, among others.

Supine Pull to Chest II

START

Lie down on your back and bend one hip and knee so that the sole of your foot contacts the floor. Bend and rotate your other hip outward as you simultaneously bend the knee on the same side; your leg will cross over the opposite leg. Hold the outside of the crossed ankle against the knee of the leg in contact with the floor. Place your hands on the sides of your lower thigh.

TECHNIQUE

Move your hands a little farther forward to grasp just below the knee the leg that is in contact with the floor. Pull on it to accentuate the internal rotation of the hip being stretched. You will feel the stretch beneath the gluteal muscles, for the piriformis is a deep muscle.

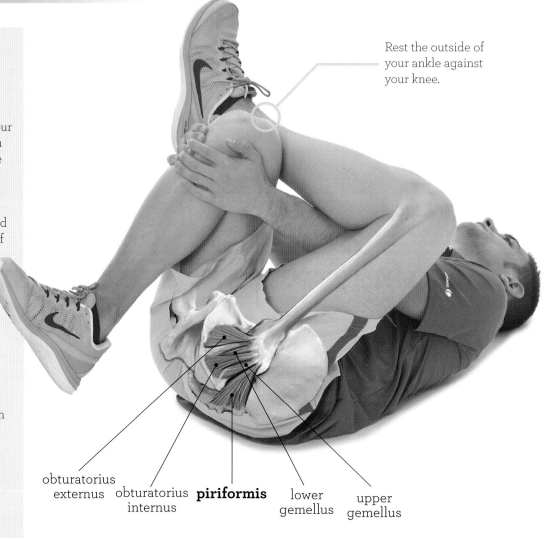

Rest the outside of your ankle against your knee.

obturatorius externus   obturatorius internus   **piriformis**   lower gemellus   upper gemellus

TENNIS	PADDLE.	SQUASH	FRONT.	BADMIN.
✔			✔	

LEVEL	SETS	DURATION
BEGINNER	2	15 s
INTERMEDIATE	2	20 s
ADVANCED	2	25 s

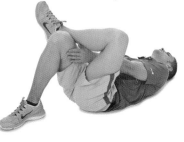

Starting Position

CAUTION

Pull carefully and in a slow, controlled manner. Keep your head on the floor, with your neck relaxed throughout the duration of this exercise.

INDICATION

For players who have experienced the piriformis syndrome or any of its symptoms, which include pain or numbness in the back of the calf, the gluteal muscles, or the lumbar region. This may be the result of the successive runs that are usual among players of racket sports.

Chair with Support

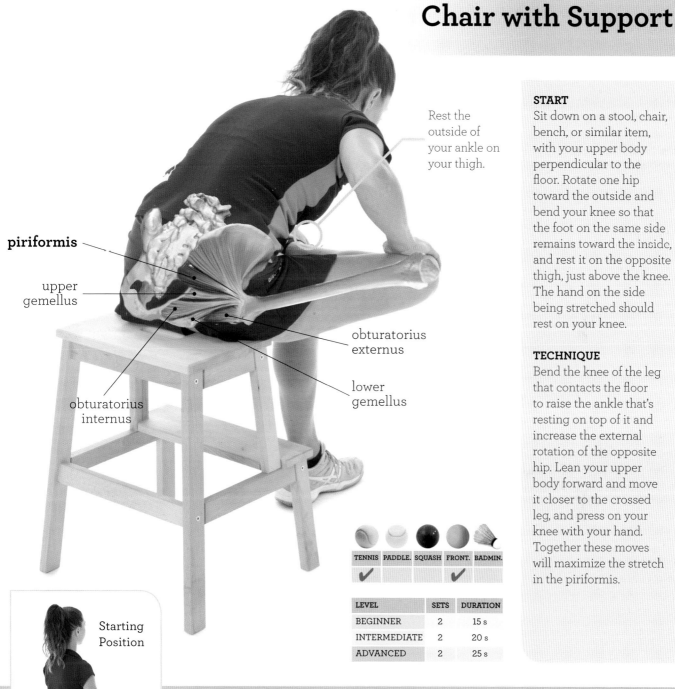

Rest the outside of your ankle on your thigh.

piriformis

upper gemellus

obturatorius internus

obturatorius externus

lower gemellus

Starting Position

TENNIS	PADDLE.	SQUASH	FRONT.	BADMIN.
✔			✔	

LEVEL	SETS	DURATION
BEGINNER	2	15 s
INTERMEDIATE	2	20 s
ADVANCED	2	25 s

START
Sit down on a stool, chair, bench, or similar item, with your upper body perpendicular to the floor. Rotate one hip toward the outside and bend your knee so that the foot on the same side remains toward the inside, and rest it on the opposite thigh, just above the knee. The hand on the side being stretched should rest on your knee.

TECHNIQUE
Bend the knee of the leg that contacts the floor to raise the ankle that's resting on top of it and increase the external rotation of the opposite hip. Lean your upper body forward and move it closer to the crossed leg, and press on your knee with your hand. Together these moves will maximize the stretch in the piriformis.

CAUTION
This stretch places significant demands on the piriformis, so you should go only as far as you feel comfortable, keeping in mind that stretching always involves a certain amount of discomfort.

INDICATION
For players who experience discomfort in the piriformis muscle due to running. This stretch helps prevent that discomfort and piriformis syndrome, which can appear as pain in the back of the thigh, the gluteal muscles, and/or the lumbar region.

LEG AND FOOT STRETCHES

The aforementioned muscles that move the knee, along with the ones that move the hip, get a lot of use in running and moving, and this includes racket and paddle sports. As a result, the knee extensor muscles may suffer strain, especially if we combine running with stopping and returns from isolated strides and/or jumping. In addition, problems may arise with the tendons responsible for straightening the knee, such as tendonitis of the quadriceps and the kneecap, when the distances covered are fairly long, as in tennis, or under fairly extreme tension as in rapid play on non-slip surfaces, as with squash. Also, the ischiotibial muscles, the knee flexors, and the hip extensors are used in running starts and jumping, so they may be affected if they are not properly developed and conditioned. The plantar flexor muscles of the ankle are used a lot in both jumping and running, and with particular intensity in running starts, a point where many injuries arise, including rupture of the middle head of the gastrocnemius, which is called "tennis leg" with good reason. The dorsal flexor muscles of the ankle obviously are used for movement in racket and paddle sports, so players are susceptible to the discomfort that is more common among runners, such as tibial periostitis (shin splints). Fibular periostitis can affect tennis players because of the demands placed on the fibular muscles by lateral moves. Finally, even the plantar aponeurosis is subjected to great tension as a result of the repeated demands on the front of the foot while running.

QUADRICEPS FEMORIS
This is the main muscle responsible for straightening the knee; it is composed of the following four muscles.
Rectus Femoris: This muscle originates at the anteroinferior iliac spine and the roof of the acetabulum, and it inserts at the tibial tuberosity through the tendon of the quadriceps femoris, the kneecap, and the patellar ligament. It shares an insertion with the vastus medialis, lateralis, and intermedialis muscles. Its main function is straightening the knee, but it also participates in bending the hip.
Vastus Lateralis: This muscle originates at the trochanter major and the lateral lip of the linea aspera of the femur, and it shares a function with the vastus medialis and intermedialis muscles in straightening the knee.
Vastus Medialis: This muscle originates at the middle lip of the linea aspera and the intertrochanteric line of the femur.
Vastus Intermedialis: This muscle originates at the antepatellar surface of the body of the femur.

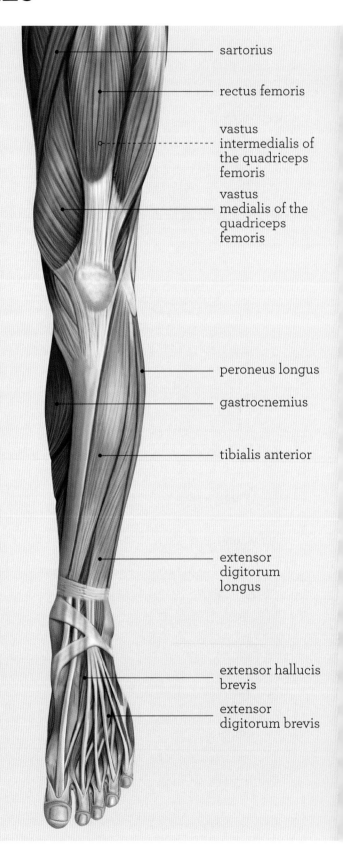

sartorius

rectus femoris

vastus intermedialis of the quadriceps femoris

vastus medialis of the quadriceps femoris

peroneus longus

gastrocnemius

tibialis anterior

extensor digitorum longus

extensor hallucis brevis

extensor digitorum brevis

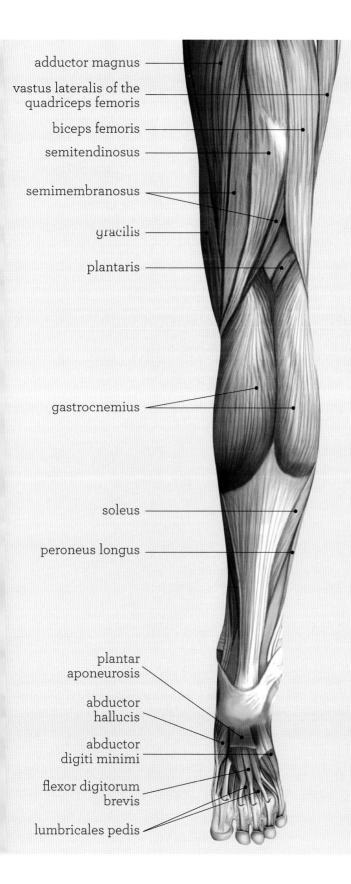

adductor magnus

vastus lateralis of the
quadriceps femoris

biceps femoris

semitendinosus

semimembranosus

gracilis

plantaris

gastrocnemius

soleus

peroneus longus

plantar
aponeurosis

abductor
hallucis

abductor
digiti minimi

flexor digitorum
brevis

lumbricales pedis

BICEPS FEMORIS

This is considered one of the ischiotibial muscles, even though this really applies only to its long head; it originates at the schiatic tuberosity, and its short head originates at the lateral lip of the linea aspera of the femur. It inserts at the head of the fibula; its main function is bending the knee, even though its long head also helps in straightening the hip.

SEMITENDINOSUS

This ischiotibial muscle originates at the sciatic tuberosity, and it inserts at the medial edge of the tibial tuberosity, the goosefoot. Its functions, which are shared with the semimembranosus, are bending the ankle and straightening the hip.

SEMIMEMBRANOSUS

This muscle shares an origin with the semitendinosus, and it inserts at the medial condyle of the tibia.

GASTROCNEMIUS

This muscle originates above the lateral and medial epicondyles of the femor, and it inserts at the calcaneal tuberosity, through the calcaneal or Achilles tendon. Its main function is plantar flexion of the ankle, but it also participates in bending the knee.

SOLEUS

This muscle originates at the rear face of the head and neck of the fibula and the soleal line of the tibia, and it shares an insertion with the gastrocnemius. Its function is plantar flexion of the ankle.

TIBIALIS ANTERIOR

This muscle originates at the tibial condyle, the proximal two thirds of the tibial diaphysis, and the interosseal membrane, and it inserts at the first cuneiform bone and the first metatarsal. Its main function is dorsal flexion of the ankle; it thus contributes shock absorption and stability of the ankle upon initial contact with the ground. It is also responsible for keeping the toes raised throughout the motion.

PLANTAR APONEUROSIS (FASCIA)

This is a tough, triangular membrane of connective tissue on the sole of the foot. It contributes to holding up the plantar arch, and it is an anchor point for several muscles. It inserts at the lower face of the heel bone and the first phalanges.

Flamingo Position with Support

START

Stand and slightly bend one hip, and to a greater degree, the knee on the same side. Hold the raised leg by the ankle using the hand that is closer. Get help from a friend or use a support you can grasp with your free hand so you can keep your balance during the entire exercise.

TECHNIQUE

Pull rearward as far as possible on the ankle you are holding; this will simultaneously produce maximum hip extension and knee bend. This will bring the back of your thigh and your calf into contact; your heel will be close to the top of your gluteal muscles, and you will easily feel the tension in the front of your thigh.

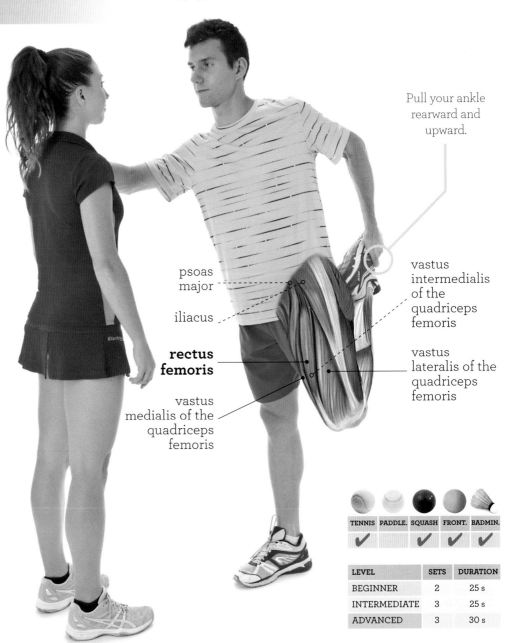

Pull your ankle rearward and upward.

psoas major

iliacus

rectus femoris

vastus medialis of the quadriceps femoris

vastus intermedialis of the quadriceps femoris

vastus lateralis of the quadriceps femoris

TENNIS	PADDLE.	SQUASH	FRONT.	BADMIN.
✔		✔	✔	✔

LEVEL	SETS	DURATION
BEGINNER	2	25 s
INTERMEDIATE	3	25 s
ADVANCED	3	30 s

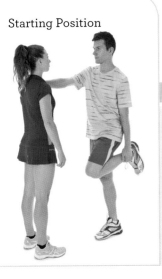

Starting Position

CAUTION

Find a friend who can help you hold the position, since it is difficult to keep your balance while doing this exercise without a support point besides your foot or the help of an assistant.

INDICATION

For athletes who experience muscle tension in the front of the thigh. Also for preventing discomfort produced by repeatedly straightening the knee against resistance, as in the jumping and running inherent in racket sports; this can entail tendonitis of the kneecap or the quadriceps, especially with play on non-slip surfaces such as wood or cement.

Knight's Position with Fitness Ball

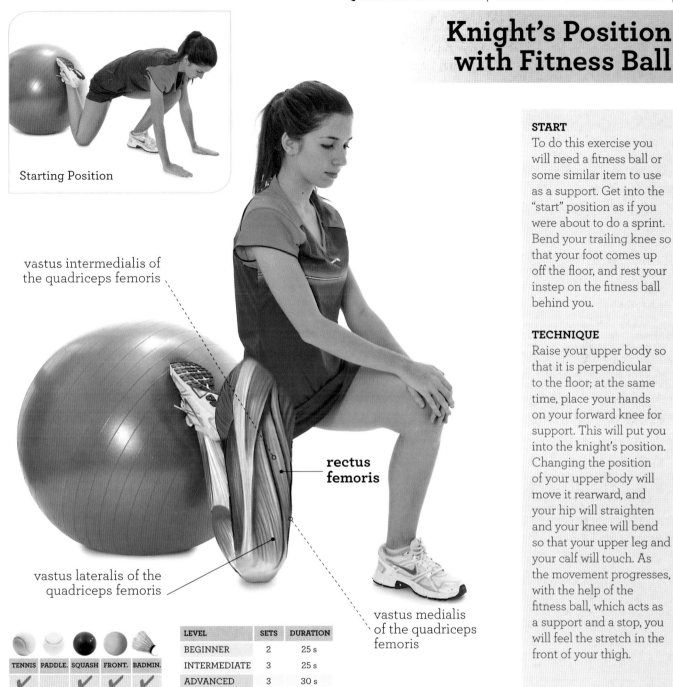

Starting Position

vastus intermedialis of the quadriceps femoris

rectus femoris

vastus lateralis of the quadriceps femoris

vastus medialis of the quadriceps femoris

LEVEL	SETS	DURATION
BEGINNER	2	25 s
INTERMEDIATE	3	25 s
ADVANCED	3	30 s

TENNIS	PADDLE.	SQUASH	FRONT.	BADMIN.
✓		✓	✓	✓

START

To do this exercise you will need a fitness ball or some similar item to use as a support. Get into the "start" position as if you were about to do a sprint. Bend your trailing knee so that your foot comes up off the floor, and rest your instep on the fitness ball behind you.

TECHNIQUE

Raise your upper body so that it is perpendicular to the floor; at the same time, place your hands on your forward knee for support. This will put you into the knight's position. Changing the position of your upper body will move it rearward, and your hip will straighten and your knee will bend so that your upper leg and your calf will touch. As the movement progresses, with the help of the fitness ball, which acts as a support and a stop, you will feel the stretch in the front of your thigh.

CAUTION

Be sure to contact the fitness ball firmly. If it moves under pressure from your foot, place it against a wall and start over. If you feel discomfort in your support knee, or if the surface is uneven, use a towel or a mat to relieve the pressure.

INDICATION

For players of racket and paddle sports because of the tension to which the hip extensor muscles are subjected in the running, jumping, and striding that these disciplines entail; also for prevention of problems such as tendonitis of the patella and quadriceps, especially if you play on surfaces with little or no slip.

Hip Extension and Assisted Knee Bend

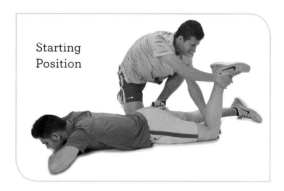

Starting Position

START

Lie face down with your legs in line with your upper body. Your helper should take a kneeling position at your side, around hip level, and hold your ankle or instep with one hand, and hold the corresponding knee with the other hand. Your partner will pull on your instep so that your knee is bent about 90°; the other hand should be on the front of your knee.

TECHNIQUE

Your helper should pull on your instep to increase the knee bend and bring your heel closer to your gluteal muscle. When your knee reaches the maximum bend, your helper will pull it upward, raising it from the floor. This will require holding your knee slightly above the kneecap.

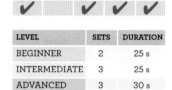

TENNIS	PADDLE.	SQUASH	FRONT.	BADMIN.
✔		✔	✔	✔

LEVEL	SETS	DURATION
BEGINNER	2	25 s
INTERMEDIATE	3	25 s
ADVANCED	3	30 s

Lift the knee from the floor.

iliacus

psoas major

vastus intermedialis of the quadriceps femoris

rectus femoris

vastus lateralis of the quadriceps femoris

vastus medialis of the quadriceps femoris

CAUTION

Communicate constantly with your helper, since this stretch is very effective; however, it is easy to go beyond the safety zone if the exercise is not done carefully and slowly.

INDICATION

For athletes who play racket and paddle sports since it helps prevent muscle discomfort and strain in the quadriceps femoris and ailments such as the tendonitis of the patella and quadriceps that are associated with jumping and running, among other movements.

Instep Pull with Exercise Band

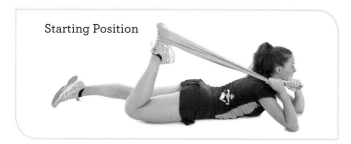

Starting Position

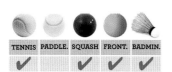

LEVEL	SETS	DURATION
BEGINNER	2	25 s
INTERMEDIATE	3	25 s
ADVANCED	3	30 s

TENNIS ✔ PADDLE. SQUASH ✔ FRONT. ✔ BADMIN. ✔

START

To do this exercise you will need a stretchable exercise band or something similar that you can use to secure onto your foot. Lie face down, bend one knee, and place the exercise band over your instep. Hold the ends of the band over your shoulder with both hands, keeping your elbows bent and without pulling on it more than necessary to keep it in place.

TECHNIQUE

Straighten your elbows, stretching the band and pulling on your instep. As you increase the intensity of the pull, your knee will bend more and your hip will extend to its limit, thereby stretching the knee extensor muscles; you will feel it in the front of your thigh.

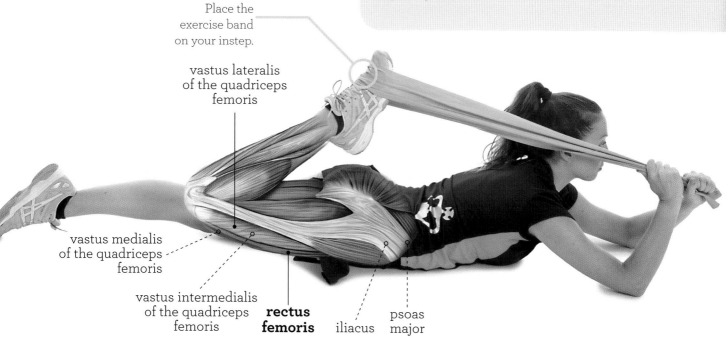

Place the exercise band on your instep.

vastus lateralis of the quadriceps femoris

vastus medialis of the quadriceps femoris

vastus intermedialis of the quadriceps femoris

rectus femoris

iliacus

psoas major

CAUTION

Make sure that the band is in good condition and held firmly in place in your hands and on your instep. Accidents are common in exercises like this one because the elastic bands break or slip off.

INDICATION

For athletes who play racket or paddle sports because of the tension to which the knee extensor muscles are subjected in jumping, running, and suddenly stopping or changing direction, among other movements, especially while playing on non-slip surfaces. This exercise helps prevent problems in the tendons of the quadriceps and the kneecap.

Standing Assisted Hip Bend

START

Stand facing a helper. Bend your hip and raise one leg, keeping your knee straight. Your helper should hold your foot with both hands under your heel and at a height where you begin to feel slight tension in the back of your thigh. Place both of your hands onto your raised thigh to make the exercise more comfortable and avoid bending your knee.

TECHNIQUE

Lean your upper body forward and increase the bend in your hip while keeping your knee totally straight; press down on your thigh with both hands to keep your knee straight. If you want to add an extra challenge, you can have your helper raise your foot slightly.

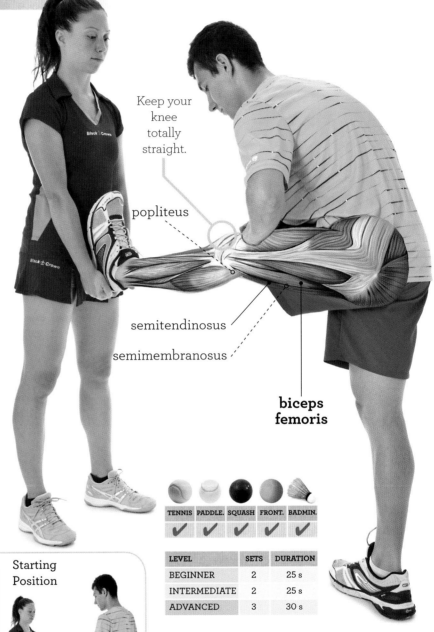

Keep your knee totally straight.

popliteus

semitendinosus

semimembranosus

biceps femoris

		TENNIS	PADDLE.	SQUASH	FRONT.	BADMIN.
		✓	✓	✓	✓	✓

LEVEL	SETS	DURATION
BEGINNER	2	25 s
INTERMEDIATE	2	25 s
ADVANCED	3	30 s

Starting Position

CAUTION

Start from a solid position and do the movements slowly so you don't lose your balance. Remember that your knee should remain straight for the exercise to be effective.

INDICATION

For athletes who play paddle or racket sports because of the demands placed on the knee flexor muscles, especially in jumps, quick starts, and sprints, and in taking long strides, especially while playing on non-slip surfaces. Also for preventing discomfort such as tendonitis of the biceps femoris, injuries to the upper thigh muscles, or tendonitis of the goosefoot.

Foot Pull with Exercise Band

Starting Position

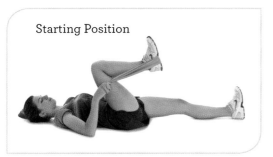

TENNIS	PADDLE.	SQUASH	FRONT.	BADMIN.
✔	✔	✔	✔	✔

LEVEL	SETS	DURATION
BEGINNER	2	25 s
INTERMEDIATE	2	25 s
ADVANCED	3	30 s

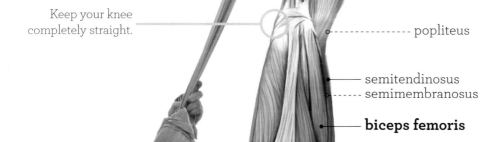

Keep your knee completely straight.

popliteus

semitendinosus
semimembranosus

biceps femoris

START
Lie down on your back with an exercise band in your hands. Bend one hip and the corresponding knee, moving your thigh toward your chest. In this position, place an exercise band on the sole of your raised foot and hold the ends in both hands, pulling only as much as you have to in order to keep the band in place.

TECHNIQUE
Straighten your knee so that the sole of your foot faces upward, and pull forcefully on the band in order to bend your hip as much as possible. Increase the intensity of the stretch by pulling harder on the exercise band; you will feel the stretch in the back of your thigh and knee.

CAUTION
Make sure that the rubber band is in good condition and secure on the sole of your foot; if it lets go, it could hit you hard in the face. Keep your head on the floor and relax your neck to avoid tension in the cervical region.

INDICATION
For athletes who play racket or paddle sports, and especially if they play on non-slip surfaces and move around a lot on the court, because of the effect of the jumps, quick starts, and sprints on the ischiotibial muscles. This stretch can protect these muscles and tendons from injuries.

Crouch with Leg Forward

START

Stand with one foot ahead of the other and your knee straight. The forward foot should rest on the heel. Bend your upper body forward and rest your hands on your thigh and near your knee.

TECHNIQUE

Lean forward with your upper body by bending at the hip of the forward leg and sliding your hands down your leg until you can touch your foot with one of them, if possible. You can rest your free hand on your knee to make sure that it stays straight and to relieve tension on your lumbar region. You will feel the tension from the stretch in the back of your thigh and knee. The opposite knee should bend slightly so that your center of gravity lowers and the bend in your hips increases.

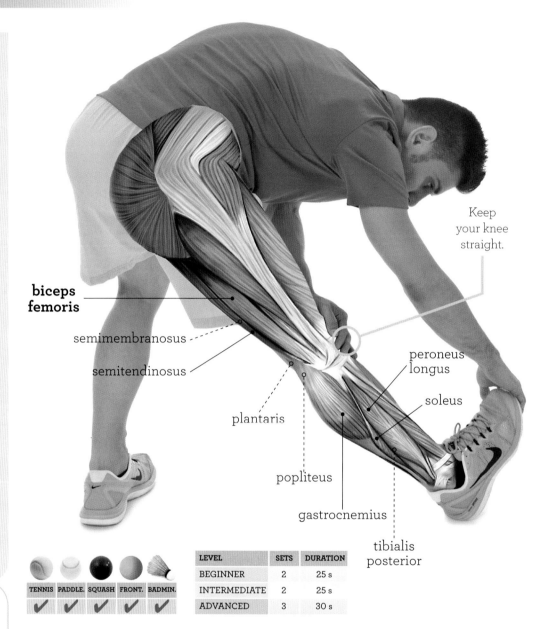

Keep your knee straight.

biceps femoris

semimembranosus

semitendinosus

plantaris

popliteus

gastrocnemius

peroneus longus

soleus

tibialis posterior

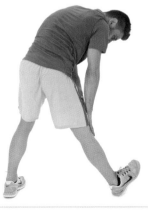

Starting Position

	TENNIS	PADDLE.	SQUASH	FRONT.	BADMIN.
	✔	✔	✔	✔	✔

LEVEL	SETS	DURATION
BEGINNER	2	25 s
INTERMEDIATE	2	25 s
ADVANCED	3	30 s

CAUTION

Start from a solid position and avoid moving downward too quickly, since the ischiotibial muscles could feel the effects. If you feel discomfort in the lumbar region, do the stretch sitting down, or prioritize keeping your lumbar spine straight rather than reaching your foot.

INDICATION

For preventing muscle and tendon discomfort in the knee flexors muscles, especially in the biceps femoris, because this muscle is used a lot in the movements inherent in racket sports, such as quick starts, running, jumping, and striding forward and back.

Seated Bilateral Hip Bend

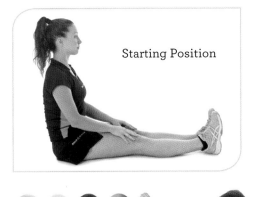

Starting Position

TENNIS	PADDLE.	SQUASH	FRONT.	BADMIN.
✔	✔	✔	✔	✔

LEVEL	SETS	DURATION
BEGINNER	2	25 s
INTERMEDIATE	3	25 s
ADVANCED	3	30 s

START
Sit down with your back and neck perpendicular to the floor, your hips bent to about a 90° angle, and your upper body and knees straight so that your heels, calves, and back of your thighs contact the floor. Rest your hands on your thighs near your knees.

TECHNIQUE
Lean your upper body forward to increase the anteversion of your pelvis and the bend in your hips. Slide your hands along your legs, trying to get as close to your feet as possible. To do this exercise properly, you should keep your knees straight during the entire movement; you will feel the tension from the stretch in the back of your thighs.

Keep your knees straight.

popliteus

biceps femoris

semitendinosus

semimembranosus

CAUTION
It's easy to reach your feet by bending your spine, but this can be bad for your intervertebral discs. Try to keep your spine in the most neutral position possible and focus on the anteversion of your pelvis, even though this means that your hands will not move as far forward.

INDICATION
For players of racket and paddle sports because of the high demands placed on the ischiotibial muscles in running, jumping, individual strides, and quick starts that are common in these disciplines. Also to prevent muscle and tendon problems, especially in athletes who play hard or on wood floors, cement, and other non-slip surfaces.

Stride with Dorsal Ankle Bend

START

Stand with your upper body erect; make sure there is enough free space ahead of you to take a long stride. Your knees should remain straight, and you can put your hands on your hips or let them hang naturally so they help you keep your balance as you do the exercise.

TECHNIQUE

Take one long stride with your forward foot, keeping the other one planted in its original position. The knee of your forward leg should bend so you can lower your center of gravity; the knee of your other leg should remain straight, with the sole of your foot, including your heel, on the floor. This will optimize the stretch, which you will feel in your calf.

Starting Position

TENNIS	PADDLE.	SQUASH	FRONT.	BADMIN.
✔	✔		✔	

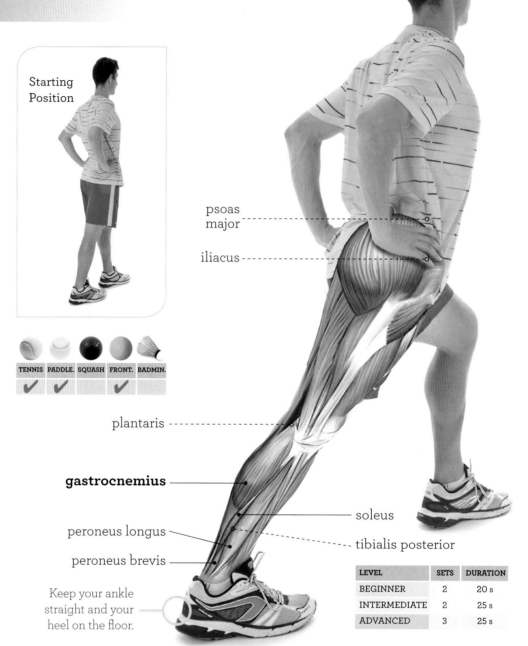

psoas major

iliacus

plantaris

gastrocnemius

soleus

peroneus longus

tibialis posterior

peroneus brevis

Keep your ankle straight and your heel on the floor.

LEVEL	SETS	DURATION
BEGINNER	2	20 s
INTERMEDIATE	2	25 s
ADVANCED	3	25 s

CAUTION

It is important to keep the heel of the leg being stretched in contact with the floor, and your knee straight while doing this exercise; this will assure proper performance of the stretch. If the tension is not sufficient after the stride, lower your center of gravity by bending the forward knee.

INDICATION

For prevention of strains in the muscles responsible for plantar ankle flexion; they do intense work in jumping and sprinting while playing paddle and racket sports. Also, along with strength work, this stretch helps prevent tennis leg or rupture of the middle head of the gastrocnemius, which is fairly common in tennis players over the age of 35.

Unilateral Pull with Exercise Band

Starting Position

TENNIS	PADDLE.	SQUASH	FRONT.	BADMIN.
✔	✔		✔	

Keep the back of your knee on the floor and your ankle in dorsal flexion.

START
Sit down with one leg drawn up and the other one straight. Keep your knee straight throughout the exercise. Place an exercise band over the sole of your foot at the level of your metatarsophalangeal joints, and hold the two ends with your hands. The tension from the band at this point is minimal; that way it will not slip off your foot. Keep your elbows straight.

TECHNIQUE
Bend your elbows and pull rearward by straightening your shoulders so that the exercise band pulls on your foot and produces dorsal ankle flexion. The harder you pull on the band, the greater the intensity of the stretch, which you will feel in your calf and the back of your knee.

LEVEL	SETS	DURATION
BEGINNER	2	20 s
INTERMEDIATE	2	25 s
ADVANCED	3	25 s

soleus

peroneus brevis

plantaris **gastrocnemius** tibialis posterior peroneus longus

CAUTION
Make sure that the exercise band is firmly in place on your foot, and that it is not old or damaged; if it breaks or slips off, it could hit you. Also keep your knee totally straight to get the most out of the exercise.

INDICATION
For relieving tension in the plantar flexor muscles of the ankle because of the demands to which they are subjected in running, jumping, and sprinting—all of which are common to the racket and paddle sports. Along with strengthening exercises, it can prevent tennis leg or rupture of the middle head of the gastrocnemius, which is common in players over the age of 35

Bilateral on Step

START

Stand next to a step or some other item of similar height that provides a firm support. Place your toes on it and keep your ankles in a neutral position or slight plantar flexion, with your knees straight. Make sure your balance is stable before you begin.

TECHNIQUE

Let your weight produce dorsal ankle flexion while you keep your knees straight. These two moves will cause your center of gravity to lower slightly and will stretch the muscles that perform plantar ankle flexion. You will feel the stretch in your calves and the back of your knees.

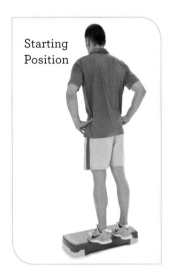

Starting Position

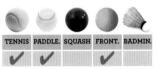

TENNIS	PADDLE.	SQUASH	FRONT.	BADMIN.
✔	✔		✔	

LEVEL	SETS	DURATION
BEGINNER	2	20 s
INTERMEDIATE	2	25 s
ADVANCED	3	25 s

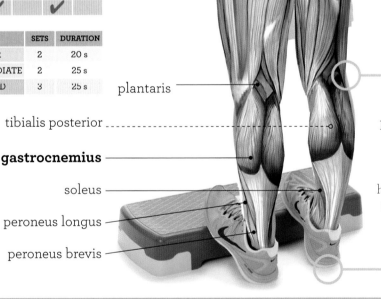

plantaris

tibialis posterior

gastrocnemius

soleus

peroneus longus

peroneus brevis

Keep your knees straight and your heels lower than your toes.

CAUTION

This exercise involves assuming an unstable position; you may prefer to use a support you can hold onto, or a friend who can help you maintain the position.

INDICATION

For relief of tension in the calf muscles; along with strengthening exercises, for preventing the strain and injury in the muscles and tendons of this area that are common to players of racket and paddle sports, which involve repeated running, fast starts, and jumps. Possible injuries include rupture of the middle head of the gastrocnemius, and inflammation of the Achilles tendon.

Assisted Dorsal Ankle Bend

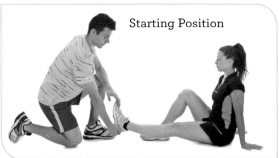

Starting Position

TENNIS	PADDLE.	SQUASH	FRONT.	BADMIN.
✔	✔		✔	

START

Sit down with one leg drawn up and the other one straight. Your friend or helper should get into the knight's position next to the foot or leg being stretched, and hold it with one hand on the heel and the other one on the toes. You should keep your knee straight and your heel slightly off the floor.

TECHNIQUE

You friend should hold your heel firmly and push your toes toward your knee; this will produce dorsal flexion in your ankle, and thus a stretch in the plantar flexor muscles. You will feel the tension from the stretch in your calf and the rear of your knee.

LEVEL	SETS	DURATION
BEGINNER	2	20 s
INTERMEDIATE	2	25 s
ADVANCED	3	25 s

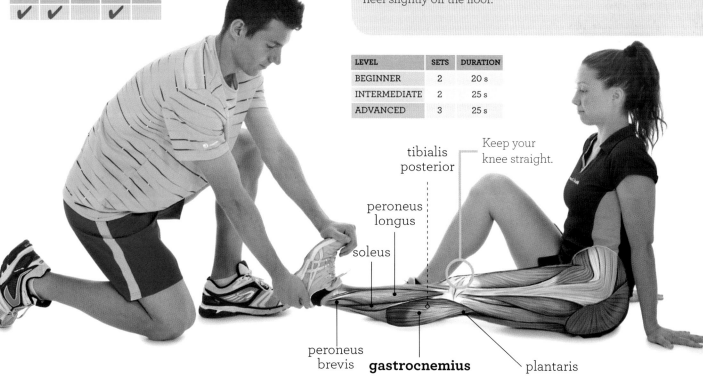

tibialis posterior

Keep your knee straight.

peroneus longus

soleus

peroneus brevis

gastrocnemius

plantaris

CAUTION

Even though you have to use considerable force in this exercise, given the strength of the muscles being stretched, you and your helper should communicate constantly to assure a risk-free stretch. You can use a rest for the ankle being stretched if that makes things easier for you.

INDICATION

Along with strengthening exercises, for preventing muscle strain and injuries to the muscles and tendons in the ankle flexor muscles, which are common among players of racket sports, such as sprints, runs, and jumps. Also for preventing typical injuries in racket and paddle sports, such as rupture of the middle head of the gastrocnemius and inflammation of the Achilles tendon.

Foot Pull on Step

START

From a standing position, place one foot on a step or other solid raised surface. Lean your upper body forward and use one hand to hold your toes up; the corresponding knee will be bent and your ankle will be in a neutral position.

TECHNIQUE

Pull upward on your toes while keeping your heel on the step and your knee bent. This move will produce dorsal ankle flexion and stretch some of the muscles used for plantar flexion. You will feel the tension in the deepest part of your calf.

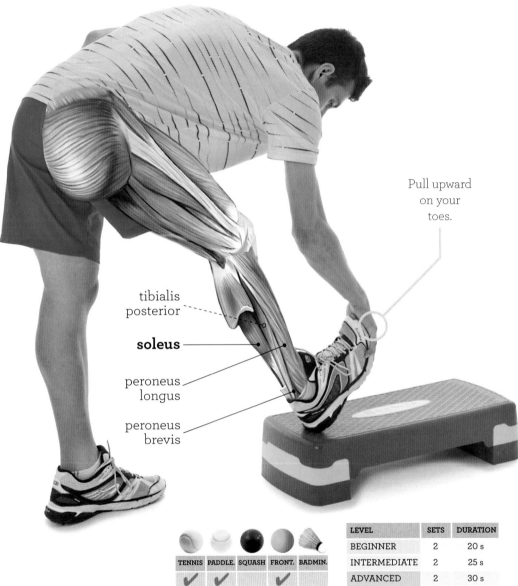

Pull upward on your toes.

tibialis posterior

soleus

peroneus longus

peroneus brevis

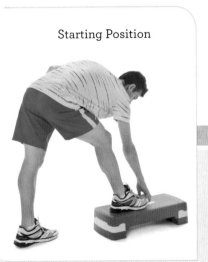

Starting Position

	TENNIS	PADDLE.	SQUASH	FRONT.	BADMIN.
	✓	✓		✓	

LEVEL	SETS	DURATION
BEGINNER	2	20 s
INTERMEDIATE	2	25 s
ADVANCED	2	30 s

CAUTION

This exercise does not involve any particular risk; you merely need to keep in mind that you can keep your knee bent slightly to affect the soleus rather than the gastrocnemius.

INDICATION

For prevention of the ailments that commonly afflict athletes in racket and paddle sports, such as tendonitis of the Achilles tendon and the tibialis posterior, as a result of quick running starts and jumping while playing these sports. These problems are fairly common in middle-aged tennis players who play fast and with greater mobility on the court.

Knee Bend with Tennis Ball

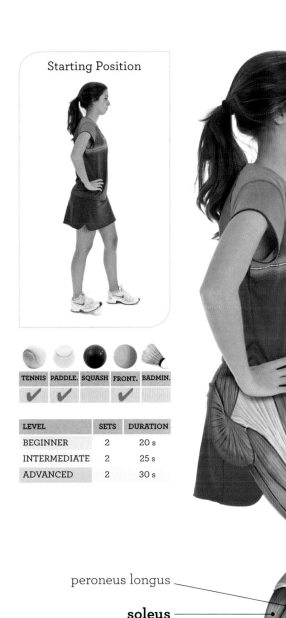

Starting Position

TENNIS	PADDLE.	SQUASH	FRONT.	BADMIN.
✔	✔		✔	

LEVEL	SETS	DURATION
BEGINNER	2	20 s
INTERMEDIATE	2	25 s
ADVANCED	2	30 s

peroneus longus

soleus

tibialis posterior

peroneus brevis

Place the ball under the front of your rear foot.

START
Stand with one foot slightly ahead of the other. Place a ball, preferably a tennis ball, paddle ball, or frontenis ball, under the front of your rear foot; this will produce a slight dorsal flexion in your ankle. Then return your upper body to vertical and place your hands on your hips.

TECHNIQUE
Bend both knees so that your center of gravity moves downward; keep your feet in their original support positions. This will accentuate the dorsal ankle flexion caused by the ball, and thus will stretch the main muscles responsible for plantar ankle flexion, except for the gastrocnemius; you will feel the tension in the deep part of your calf.

CAUTION

Even though this exercise involves no risk, be careful to center the ball under your foot so that there is adequate movement in your ankle. If you use a tennis ball or a paddle ball it will be easier to do the exercise on a rough surface.

INDICATION

For prevention of ailments common to players of racket sports, such as tendonitis in the tibialis posterior and the Achilles tendon, which commonly results from quick starts, running, and jumping; these problems occur more frequently with fast or long runs and prolonged or frequent play.

Step Support and Knee Bend

START

Take a position on a step by resting on your toes; have your helper face you close enough so you can rest your hands on his shoulders. Your helper should also hold you for greater stability while performing the stretch. Lift one leg by bending your hip and knee, and rest your instep on the back of your other leg.

TECHNIQUE

Relax the muscles that perform plantar ankle flexion, allowing your ankle to gradually sag into dorsal flexion; this will lower your center of gravity. To this movement add a slight bend in your support knee in order to minimize the involvement of your gastrocnemius. You will feel the tension from the muscle stretch in the deep part of your calf.

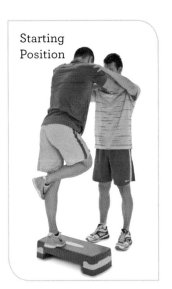

Starting Position

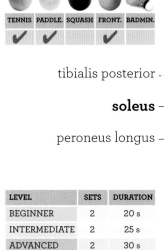

TENNIS	PADDLE.	SQUASH	FRONT.	BADMIN.
✔	✔		✔	

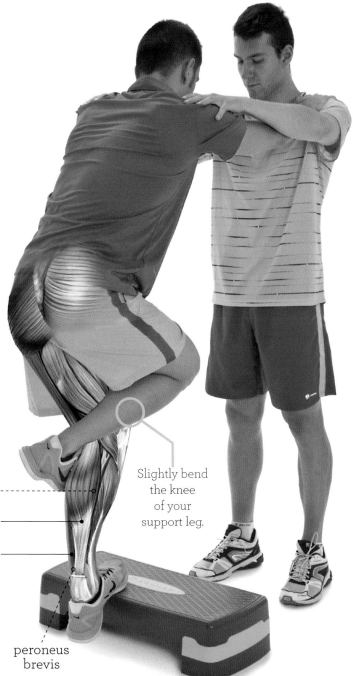

tibialis posterior

soleus

peroneus longus

peroneus brevis

Slightly bend the knee of your support leg.

LEVEL	SETS	DURATION
BEGINNER	2	20 s
INTERMEDIATE	2	25 s
ADVANCED	2	30 s

CAUTION

Given the inherently unstable position used in this exercise, try to use a support that remains immovable even with all your weight on the edge, and get help from an assistant so you can do it without interruption to adjust your balance.

INDICATION

For prevention of muscle strain and tendonitis in the tibialis posterior and the Achilles tendon; these commonly occur as the result of quick starts, running, and jumping. All these actions are used while playing paddle and racket sports, and they occur more frequently in athletes who play long matches or ones that involve long, fast running.

To the Rear on All Fours

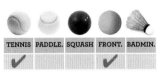

Starting Position

TENNIS	PADDLE.	SQUASH	FRONT.	BADMIN.
✔			✔	

LEVEL	SETS	DURATION
BEGINNER	2	20 s
INTERMEDIATE	2	25 s
ADVANCED	2	25 s

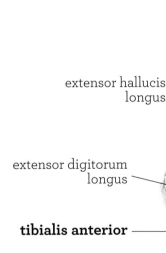

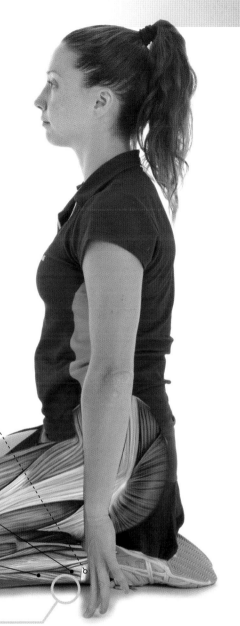

third peroneus

extensor hallucis longus

extensor digitorum longus

tibialis anterior

Try to keep your insteps and shins in line.

START
Get down on all fours with your hands in line with your shoulders, your knees together, and your heels under your gluteal muscles. Your feet should rest on your toes, and your ankles should be in a nearly neutral position. Your hips will bend at about a 45° angle, and your knees will be nearly completely bent, so you will almost be touching your heels.

TECHNIQUE
Bend your knees all the way, slide your hands to the rear, and straighten your upper body so that you are sitting on your heels. This will produce total plantar flexion of your ankles and stretch the muscles that are used in the opposite action. You will feel the stretch in the front of your legs and ankles.

CAUTION
Because of the pressure applied to your ankles as this exercise progresses, you should do the stretch slowly and maintain slight pressure on your hands throughout. These precautions will make it easier for you to hold the stretch and relieve the pressure on your ankles if you feel any discomfort.

INDICATION
For relief of muscle tension in the front of the leg and prevention of problems such as shin splints, which affects mainly runners, but also athletes whose disciplines involve running; this is the case in most racket sports, particularly on hard surfaces.

Dance Step

START

Stand with one foot ahead of the other at a distance slightly greater than one normal step. Your upper body should be perpendicular to the floor; your arms can hang relaxed by your body, or you can place your hands on your hips or thighs if that is more comfortable or more stable.

TECHNIQUE

Move your center of gravity forward and lower it slightly while keeping your upper body erect. Support most of your weight on your forward foot and bend your knee a little. Your trailing foot will have to gradually come off the floor until it makes contact only with your toes. Your ankle will be in plantar flexion with your instep facing downward. Try to maximize the plantar flexion to get the most out of the stretch.

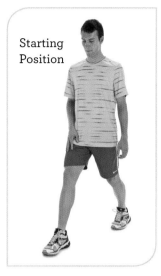

Starting Position

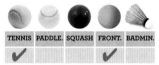

	TENNIS	PADDLE.	SQUASH	FRONT.	BADMIN.
	✔		✔		

LEVEL	SETS	DURATION
BEGINNER	2	20 s
INTERMEDIATE	2	25 s
ADVANCED	2	30 s

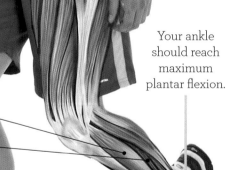

tibialis anterior

extensor digitorum longus

extensor hallucis longus

third peroneus

Your ankle should reach maximum plantar flexion.

CAUTION

This exercise presents no significant risks since the joints are not subjected to excessive pressure, and muscle tension is moderate. The only thing you need to pay attention to is keeping your balance as you move your weight toward the front support.

INDICATION

For players who feel muscle tension in the front of the leg or who want to prevent certain ailments caused by running, such as tibial periostitis (shin splints); this occurs more frequently in athletes who play on hard surfaces or run long distances.

Seated with Leg on Thigh

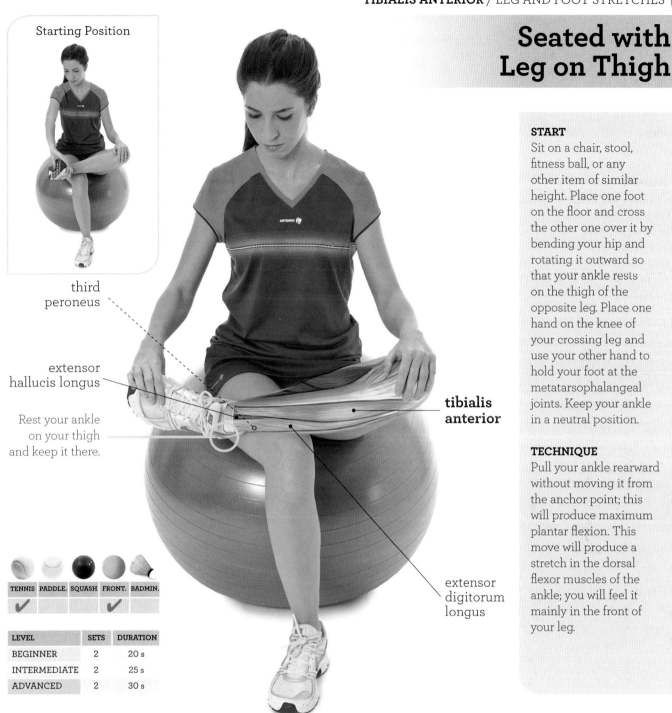

Starting Position

third peroneus

extensor hallucis longus

Rest your ankle on your thigh and keep it there.

tibialis anterior

extensor digitorum longus

	TENNIS	PADDLE.	SQUASH	FRONT.	BADMIN.
	✔			✔	

LEVEL	SETS	DURATION
BEGINNER	2	20 s
INTERMEDIATE	2	25 s
ADVANCED	2	30 s

START

Sit on a chair, stool, fitness ball, or any other item of similar height. Place one foot on the floor and cross the other one over it by bending your hip and rotating it outward so that your ankle rests on the thigh of the opposite leg. Place one hand on the knee of your crossing leg and use your other hand to hold your foot at the metatarsophalangeal joints. Keep your ankle in a neutral position.

TECHNIQUE

Pull your ankle rearward without moving it from the anchor point; this will produce maximum plantar flexion. This move will produce a stretch in the dorsal flexor muscles of the ankle; you will feel it mainly in the front of your leg.

CAUTION

Hold the leg being stretched in order to limit the ankle movement and keep other joints from absorbing the pull and reducing the effectiveness of the exercise. Be sure to hold your foot correctly and avoid pulling it by the toes.

INDICATION

For players who feel abnormal muscle tension in the front of the leg, or who want to prevent tibial periostitis (shin splints), which often results from extended running, especially on hard surfaces, with improper footwear, and from fairly long total distances covered.

Inversion with Support

START

Stand with your feet parallel and shoulder width apart. Keep your upper body perpendicular to the floor, your knees straight, and your toes pointing straight forward. You can put your hands on your hips for comfort, but they will not be called on to perform any action.

TECHNIQUE

Place the foot being stretched in inversion so that the contact is along its side, and move your center of gravity slightly toward this side so that your body weight adds to the inversion. You will feel very slight tension, if you feel anything at all, in the side of your foot.

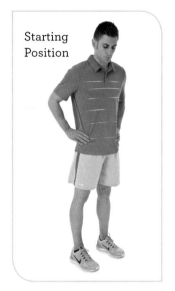

Starting Position

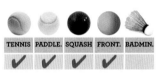

TENNIS	PADDLE.	SQUASH	FRONT.	BADMIN.
✔	✔	✔	✔	

LEVEL	SETS	DURATION
BEGINNER	2	15 s
INTERMEDIATE	2	20 s
ADVANCED	2	25 s

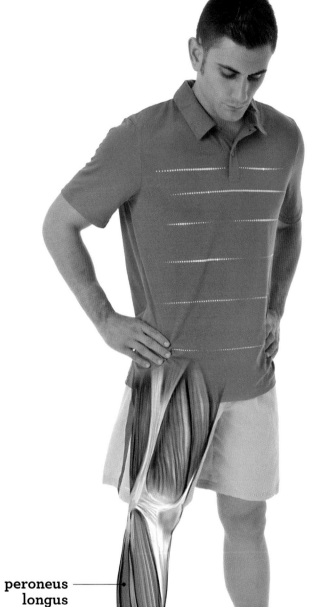

peroneus longus

peroneus brevis

third peroneus

Rest your foot along the outside.

CAUTION

This exercise places weight on your ankle in an abnormally weak position, so you should perform the inversion movement slowly and return to the starting position before you feel any discomfort that does not belong in a stretch.

INDICATION

Along with strengthening exercises, for prevention of peroneal tendonitis and other ailments that are commonly associated with the lateral moves that are inherent in paddle and racket sports.

Seated Ankle Inversion

TENNIS	PADDLE.	SQUASH	FRONT.	BADMIN.
✔	✔	✔	✔	

LEVEL	SETS	DURATION
BEGINNER	2	15 s
INTERMEDIATE	2	20 s
ADVANCED	2	25 s

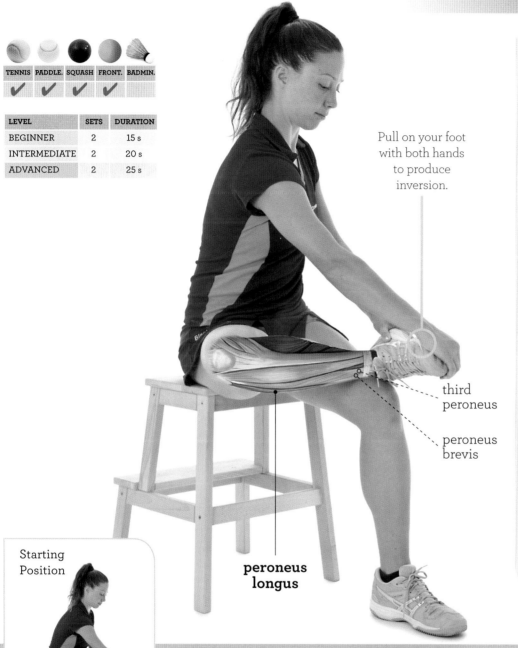

Pull on your foot with both hands to produce inversion.

third peroneus

peroneus brevis

peroneus longus

Starting Position

START

Sit on a chair or a stool, rest one foot on the floor, and cross one leg over the other by bending your hip and rotating it outward. The outside of your ankle should rest on the lower part of the opposite thigh. Hold the heel of the foot being stretched with one hand and the front part with the other.

TECHNIQUE

Pull on your foot with both hands to produce inversion; keep your ankle resting on the opposite thigh. You will feel very subtle tension in the outside of your leg; you may not even feel like you are stretching, like when you are working your hip adductor muscles or your ischiotibial muscles.

CAUTION

Proceed cautiously, and avoid continually increasing the strength of your pull. Remember that in this case the absence of muscle tension does not mean that you are doing the exercise improperly.

INDICATION

Along with strengthening exercises, for prevention of pereoneal tendonitis; this condition commonly affects players of paddle and racket sports because of the repeated lateral moves; also for alleviating abnormal tension in the muscles used for foot eversion.

Foot Rolls with Tennis Ball

START

When you do this exercise it's a good idea to take off your shoes to improve the pressure and the stretch on the sole of your foot. Stand with a ball under the front of your foot, preferably a tennis, paddle, or frontenis ball, because of their greater size. Keep your spine erect and use your arms for balance if necessary.

TECHNIQUE

Slide your foot forward so that the ball rolls between the floor and the sole of your foot. When the ball is below the arch of your foot, increase the pressure as if you were trying to deform the ball. You can move your foot an inch or so forward and back on the ball to cover more of the plantar aponeurosis (fascia).

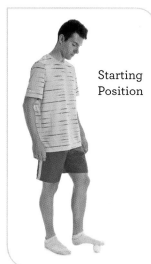

Starting Position

	TENNIS	PADDLE.	SQUASH	FRONT.	BADMIN.
	✓	✓		✓	✓

LEVEL	SETS	DURATION
BEGINNER	2	25 s
INTERMEDIATE	3	25 s
ADVANCED	3	30 s

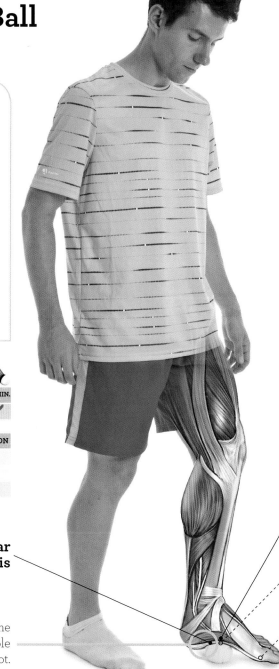

plantar aponeurosis

flexor digitorum brevis

quadratus plantae

abductor hallucis

Press down on the ball with the sole of your foot.

CAUTION

This exercise involves no risks, but it's a good idea to use balls that offer a certain amount of resistance to deformation, without being too hard, in order to optimize the results of the stretch. You can use any kind of ball on a rough surface, but it is best not to use felt-covered balls on smooth surfaces.

INDICATION

For prevention of plantar fasciitis, which is caused by repeated pressure and tension on the plantar aponeurosis (fascia); this can affect people who play racket and paddle sports because of the tension on the sole of the foot produced by running and jumping, especially if proper footwear is not used.

Toe Pull

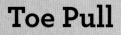

Starting Position

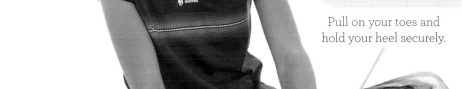

TENNIS	PADDLE.	SQUASH	FRONT.	BADMIN.
✔	✔	✔	✔	

START

Sit down, stretch out one leg, and cross the other one over the opposite thigh by using external rotation of your thigh and bending your knee. The crossing leg will rest on the opposite thigh, and you will have to take off your shoe to work on your toes. Hold your heel with one hand and your toes with the other one.

TECHNIQUE

Pull on your toes to straighten your metatarsophalangeal joints; keep your ankle in place and continue to hold your heel. You will note that the sole of your foot tenses and hardens to the touch, mainly as a result of stretching the plantar aponeurosis and the short flexor muscle of the toes.

Pull on your toes and hold your heel securely.

flexor digitorum brevis

abductor hallucis

plantar aponeurosis

quadratus plantae

LEVEL	SETS	DURATION
BEGINNER	2	15 s
INTERMEDIATE	2	20 s
ADVANCED	2	25 s

CAUTION

Be careful when you pull on your toes, and remember that the interphalangeal joints are particularly fragile, so they should not be subjected to the bulk of the pulling force. If you feel any discomfort or pain in your joints, reduce the force.

INDICATION

For prevention of plantar fasciitis, which is common in sports that involve running, such as racket and paddle sports. This malady is due to the repeated tension endured by the plantar aponeurosis (fascia) in successive strides, particularly if proper footwear is not used.

Alphabetical Index of Muscles

obliques, 23–25, 28

obturatorius externus, 123–125

obturatorius internus, 108, 123–125

omohyoid, 8

palmaris longus, 8, 90, 98–99, 102–103

pectineus, 8, 42, 44, 117–19

pectoralis major, 8, 23–25, 36–39, 62, 72, 74–76, 81–85, 88, 90, 92, 93–94

pectoralis minor, 72, 86

peroneus brevis, 47, 136–142, 146–147

peroneus longus, 9, 47, 126–127, 134, 136–142, 146–47

peroneus muscles, 30, 146–147

piriformis, 108, 113–115, 123–125

plantar aponeurosis, 31, 126–127, 148–149

plantar flexion, 6–7, 10–11, 30, 45, 65, 127, 138, 140, 143–145

plantaris, 9, 127, 134, 136–139

popliteus, 132–135

posterior scalene, 56–57

pronator teres, 90

psoas major, 43, 46, 67–68, 108–112, 128, 130–131, 136

psoas minor, 67–68, 109–112

quadratus femoris, 108

quadratus lumborum, 41, 52, 69–71

quadratus plantae, 148–149

quadriceps femoris, 8–9, 29, 46, 126–131

rectus abdominis, 8, 23–28, 41, 52–53, 67–68, 71

rectus femoris, 126, 128–131

rhomboid, 23–25, 38, 52, 54–55

rhomboideus major, 38, 52–55, 61, 73, 78, 89

rhomboideus minor, 38, 52–55, 61, 73, 78, 89

rotator, shoulder, 23–26, 76, 78–81

rotator cuff, 27, 77–79

rotators, 53, 60–65, 78, 79–81

sartorius, 8, 52, 126

scalene, 8, 56–57, 72

scalenus anterior, 56–57, 72

scalenus medius, 56–57, 72

scalenus posterior, 56–57

semimembranosus, 9, 43, 108, 127, 132–135

semispinalis, 52–53, 55, 58–59

semispinalis thoracis, 60–65, 64

semitendinosus, 9, 43, 108, 127, 132–135

serratus anterior, 8, 23–25, 28, 36–39, 52, 72–73, 86–87, 90

soleus, 8–9, 30, 47, 127, 134, 136–142

spinalis thoracis, 60–65

splenius capitis, 9, 53, 58–59, 73

splenius cervicis, 58–59

sternocleidomastoid, 8–9, 57, 59, 72

subscapularis, 72–73, 80–81

supraspinatus, 53, 73, 75, 78–79

tensor fasciae latae, 8–9, 44, 52–53, 108–109, 120–122

teres major, 9, 25, 37, 39–40, 53, 63, 73, 80–81, 87–88, 95–97

teres minor, 9, 53, 63, 72, 73, 77–79, 89

third peroneus, 6–7, 143–147

thoracic iliocostalis, 52, 55, 60, 62–63

thoracic spine, 60–61

tibialis anterior, 6–8, 126–127, 143–145

tibialis posterior, 30, 47, 134, 136, 138–142

trapezius, 8–9, 23–25, 38, 40, 52–56, 66–69, 72–73

triceps brachii, 8–9, 23, 25, 53, 73, 90–91, 95–97

upper gemellus, 108, 113–115, 123–125

vastus intermedius, 48, 126, 128–131

vastus lateralis, 48, 126, 128–131

vastus medialis, 48, 126, 128–131

Bibliography

Benno, M. *Injury and Performance on Tennis Surfaces.* University of Calgary, 2003

Chard, M.D.; Lahman, S.M. "Racket Sports—Patterns of Injury Presenting to a Sports Injury Clinic." [sic] *British Journal of Sports Medicine* 1987; 21: 150–153

Der Hoeven, Hvan; Kibler, W.B. "Shoulder Injuries in Tennis Players." *British Journal of Sports Medicine,* 2006; 40: 435–550

Ellenbecker, Todd; Pluim, Babette; Vivier, Stephane; Sniteman, Clay. *Common Injuries in Tennis Players: Exercises to Address Muscular Imbalance and Reduce Injury Risk.* National Strength and Conditioning Association, 2009; 31 (4)

Gallo, Robert A. *Tennis Injuries.* Sports Medicine (American Orthopedic Society for Sports Medicine), 2010

Gerard, Olivier; Eicher, F. Micallef, J.P.; Millet, G.P. "Effects of the Playing Surface on Plantar Pressures and Potential Injuries in Tennis." *British Journal of Sports Medicine* 2006; 41; 733–738

Kibler, W. Ben; Brody, Howard; Knudson, Duane; Stroia, Kathleen. *Tennis Technique and Injury Prevention.* Usta Sport Science Committee White Paper, 2014

Kolowich, Patricia. *Tennis Injuries.* American Orthopedic Society for Sports Medicine, 2010

Kor, Alex. *Doubles Partners: Common Lower Extremity Tennis Injuries.* American Academy of Pediatric Sports Medicine 2011; 91–98

Madden, Christopher; Putukian, Margot; McCarty, Eric; Young, C. Craig. *Netter's Sport Medicine.* Elsevier, 2009